PUBLIC HEALTH AND HOMOEOPATHY FOR HIV IN INDIA

BY

Edward J. Mills

B. Jain Publishers (P) Ltd.
New Delhi

Note

Any information given in this book is not intended to be taken as a replacement for medical advice. Any person with a condition requiring medical attention should consult a qualified practitioner or therapist.

First edition : 2000

All rights are reserved. No part of this publication may be reproduced, stored in a retrieval system or transmitted, in any form or by any means, mechanical, recording or otherwise, without prior written permission of the publishers

Price : Rs. 95/-

© Copyright Reserved

Published by :
Kuldeep Jain
For

B. Jain Publishers (P.) Ltd.

1921, Street No.10, Chuna Mandi
Paharganj, New Delhi-110 055 (INDIA)
Phones: 3670430; 3670572; 3683100, 3683200, 3683300
FAX : 011-3610471 & 3683400
Email : bjain@vsnl.com
Website : www.bjainindia.com

Printed in India by:
Unisons Techno Financial Consultants (P) Ltd.
522, FIE, Patpar Ganj, Delhi- 110 092.

ISBN : 81-7021-1010-4
BOOK CODE : BM-5452

Acknowledgements

My utmost appreciation goes to Dr. Cory Ross, the program coordinator at The Canadian College of Naturopathic Medicine for having faith when I had lost mine.

Thanks to Ms. Penny Tantakis for giving me the chance to learn.

My sincerest gratitude to Dr. Kaushal Jain of Baroda, Gujarat, for standing up against all those who said "he shouldn't do it" and accepting and specializing in HIV treatment. Dr. Jain allowed me to observe many of his patients and see the difference that his treatment made.

The entire staff of the Emery Hospital in Anand, Gujarat, for loving and dedicating their lives to others. I owe them so much.

To the entire staff of the Salvation Army HIV/AIDS team in Byculla, Mumbai; against an enormous challenge; they went on steadfast. Particular thanks to Dr. Nagesh Shirgoppiker; if only there were more progressive thinkers like him.

Dr. Pankaj Dave, who challenged me to dedicate myself to this field. I have much admiration for his knowledge and progressive thinking.

To the entire staff of the Homoeopathic clinic of Dr. F. Master. I sincerely thank him for inspiring me and consistently amazing me.

To Dr. Ken Luby N.D., "thank you for all the herculean work that you have done before me and for standing strong all the time."

Many thanks to Dr. Praful Barvalia, Dr. Dilip Dikshit, Dr. Graham Baldwin, Dr. William Gapen, and to Mike Strange for all their help and inspiration.

Thanks also to George Vithoulkas for allowing the use of his insight in Materia Medica.

To Lisa, who was willing to sacrifice so much for this book, "thank you".

Finally a special thanks to Dr. Farokh J. Master M.D. (Hom.) whom taught me how to look at life, work, and the world around me. This is humbly dedicated to you.

" Man is protected from sickness in two ways, by Homoeopathy and by use. The physician and the nurse who go into the district of yellow fever or typhoid or diphtheria or smallpox, who keep busy, who have, in the highest sense of the word, the true love of the use, who have gone into the work as mediums of mercy, will largely be protected just simply from their love of the work, from their delight in it. They have no fear. Fear is an overwhelming cause of sickness; those who fall prey to fear are likely to become sick, but those who face disease with no fear are likely to remain well; they do sometimes fall sick, it is true, but I believe it is because they begin to have fear in the work."

James Tyler Kent

ABSTRACT

As the pandemic HIV/AIDS progresses relentlessly, the primary focus has been on prevention rather than treatment. The available chemotherapeutic drugs are largely unaffordable throughout the world. Therefore, an examination of principle cost- effective and result oriented therapies began in July 1999 in India.

India has the largest population of HIV+ve individuals in the world, whilst the disease is largely overlooked by the medical establishment. It is, therefore, the purpose of this paper to suggest guidelines for the treatment of individuals and the education of the population at large to prevent the spread of disease and also the social stigma attached with this disorder. Both rural communities (Gujarat) and urban (Mumbai) have been considered.

The examination indicated that homoeopathy could play a significant role in slowing down the progression of AIDS, whilst also remaining affordable even in remote rural areas. Consequently, a focus on the suggestive use of homoeopathy has been achieved.

PREFACE

The project that is included in the following pages was conducted in India between 1999 and the year 2000. The first portion of this book focuses on Public Health issues regarding the education of the population and medical community, and the acceptance of people living with HIV and AIDS. The latter portion of the book deals with the homoeopathic approach to case-taking and prescribing in HIV. These recommendations are based on the observations of many physicians all over India.

The aim of this book is not to become a text source for treatment, but rather to stimulate interest and compassion for the treatment of this disease. It has often been my observation that we must reread what we know about this disease and forget what bias we have developed as a result of hearsay . Homoeopathy has much to offer individuals diagnosed as HIV+, and treatment commencing during the asymptomatic period may be able to provide good health for years to come. It is most certainly my opinion that constitutional treatment can provide the best results, particularly during the asymptomatic periods. Of course, the experience of the physician will often determine what approach is required in a case.

Many hypothesize a cure for this disease through homoeopathy. In all of my investigations, I have never seen an individual turn seronegative. I wish that we could perform miracles like that, but we will have to settle for smaller miracles.

"To save life doomed to be lost is Divine

To save life diseases beyond repair is Superhuman.

To make an attempt to save is Human"—*Make it more clear*

[1]Master. F. J.

Contents

Chapter-1

INTRODUCTION 1
1.1 Problem Statement 1
        Table 1 : HIV Infection First Reported by Countries 2
        Table 2 : Global Trend of HIV Infection in 1999 3
1.2 Historical Approach 4

Chapter-2

DISEASE 7
2.1 Mode of Transmission 7
        Table 3 : Indian Trend of HIV infection in 1998 8
2.2 Incubation Period 9
2.3 AIDS Related Complex (ARC) or Middle
     Stage HIV Infection: 10
2.4 Acquired Immuno Deficiency Syndrome (AIDS) 11
        Table 4 : Diseases Indicating AIDS, Without
        Laboratory Findings 11
        Table 5 : WHO Clinical Case Definition (for use
        when diagnostic tools are limited) 12
        Table 6 : Opportunistic Infections 13
2.5 Screening 14
2.6 Monitoring 15

Chapter-3

EPIDEMIOLOGY 17

3.1	Epidemiological Features	17
	Table 7 : Epidemiological Model	17
3.2	Agent	18
	Table 8 : Epidemiological factors	19
3.3	Host	21

Chapter-4

ENVIRONMENT 23

4.1	HIV in India	23
4.2	Opportunistic Infections	31
4.3	Indian AIDS History	32
4.4	Case Example #1	33
4.5	Case Example #2	34
4.6	Case Example #3	35
4.7	Case Example #4	35
4.8	Case Example #5	36

Chapter-5

DEMOGRAPHICS 37

5.1	Demographics	37
5.2	Migration and Employment	37
	Table 9 : Rising Incidence of HIV in Commercial Sex Workers, 1987-1997, Mumbai	39
	Table 10 : Physical and Social Risk Factors of Poor ...	40
5.3	Women	41
	Table 11 : Rising Incidence of HIV in Women Attending Antenatal Clinics 1990- 1997, Mumbai	42
5.4	Ethics	43

Chapter-6

INFORMATION, EDUCATION, COMMUNICATION, COMPASSION. 47

- 6.1 Group I, Professional (Page-41) 47
- 6.2 Group II, General Population (Page-42) 47
- 6.3 Group III, Vulnerable Groups (Page-43) 47
- 6.4 Group IV, High Risk Groups (Page-44) 47
- 6.5 Group V, HIV+ and AIDS patients ("-45) 47
  - Table : Group I, Professional 48
  - Table : Group II, General Population 49
  - Table : Group III, Vulnerable Groups 50
  - Table : Group IV, High Risk Groups 51
  - Table : Group V, HIV+ and AIDS patients 52
- 6.6 Positive Media 53

Chapter-7

EMPOWERMENT 55

- 7.1 Positive + People 55
- 7.2 Familial Empowerment 57
- 7.5 Survey 1 61
  - Table 12 : Survey 1 : General Population 61
- 7.6 Survey 2: HIV+ve individuals 63
  - Table 13 : HIV+ Individuals 64

Chapter-8

TREATMENT 67

- 8.1 Conventional/Allopathic Medicine 67
- 8.2 Ayurvedic Medicine 69
  - Table 14 : Antiretroviral Therapy 70

8.3 Homoeopathy 72
      Table 15 : Descriptive Characteristics at the end
      of CCRH Double Blind Study 75

Chapter-9

HOMOEOPATHY 79

9.1 Indications for homoeopathic observations 79
9.2 Selecting the remedy 81
9.3 Prescribing 83
9.4 Potency 87

Chapter-10

MIASMS 89

10.1 Theory 89
10.2 Understanding the Miasmatic Picture Dominant and Fundamental Miasms 91
10.3 Dominant Miasms 92
10.4 Remedies to be considered in the psoric state: 94
10.6 Stage II: (Sycosis) (Disordered Kapha) 96
10.7 Remedies to be considered 97
10.9 Stage III: (Tubercular) (Disordered Vata Kapha) 99
10.10 Remedies to be considered in the tubercular stage: 101
10.11 Diet 101
10.12 Stage IV: (Syphilitic) (Disordered Pitta) 103
10.13 List of anti- syphilitic remedies to consider: 104
10.14 Combination Therapy: 104

Chapter-11

COST 107

11.1 Cost 107
11.2 Eradication 107

Chapter-12
PROPOSAL TO NATIONAL HIV TEAM 109
12.1 Proposal 109
12.2 Objective 109
12.3 Reason 109
12.4 Method 110
12.5 Cost 112
12.6 Time Schedule 112

Chapter-13
CONCLUSION 115

Photographic Codocil 117

Annexture-i
CASE STUDY 129
Table 1.1: Participants in study, age and sex distribution: 133
Table 1.2: Mode of infection relative to participants. 134
Table 2.1: Health status at conclusion of study, including duration of treatment. 138
Table 2.2 141
Table 2.3 141

Annexture-ii
MATERIA MEDICA 145

Annexture-iii
THEMES 185

Annexture-iv
CASE EXAMPLES 193

Annexture-v
HOMOEOPATHY IN INDIA 203

Appendix-i
BIBLIOGRAPHY 207

Appendix-ii
ENDNOTES 211

Chapter 1

INTRODUCTION

1.1 Problem Statement

The pandemic of Human Immuno Deficiency Syndrome (HIV) and Acquired Immuno Deficiency Syndrome (AIDS) has not been limited to nationality, sex, age, and socioeconomic status. HIV, the retrovirus causing AIDS has infected tens of millions of people worldwide, in developed and developing nations. The disease is truly pandemic as no continents are spared. Although AIDS was first recognized in San Francisco in 1981, earlier cases have been discovered using retrospective analysis to have occurred in Canada in 1979[i], and further back in Africa[ii]. The fact that symptoms of AIDS are usually the initial indicator of HIV infection would lead us to believe that the number of AIDS cases presently noted is but a fraction of things to come. The real measure of the disease is the number of people infected with HIV; which we will never be able to fully know as mass screening is likely impossible, due to cultural and financial restraints[iii].

Now that nineteen years have passed since the discovery[iv], the pandemic proceeds relentlessly. Up until 1999, 43'347 cases exist in Canada[v], while numbers soar in countries where the risk factor of promiscuity may be more acceptable, such as in Sub- Saharan Africa[vi] where the incidence is surpassing 1'814 per 100'000[vii] and may be as high as 30% in Zaire[viii]. Many countries, where the diagnosis of HIV infection would result in stigmatizing and nonacceptance, such as India, there are many in individuals refraining from testing to avoid the diagnosis[ix].

While public education in several countries, such as Canada, has begun to reduce the incidence[x], the HIV infection still thrives in areas where literacy and access to information are compromised. High rates of HIV infection are now reaching new communities and countries, often with great rapidity. The explosion of HIV has only recently reached South East Asia, particularly in Thailand, Burma, and India[xi]; all of which have thriving and legalized sex industries. It can be assumed that AIDS did not, in fact, only arrive in Asia during the late eighties, rather that public and medical ignorance, allowed the progression of infection to go unchecked. HIV is now reaching as remote areas as Fiji, Papua New Guinea, and Samoa. It is likely that this infection will have massive global implications affecting not only the physical and psychological status of populations, but also leading to significant economic devastation.

Table 1. HIV Infection First Reported by Countries

Country	Year	Country	Year
Bangladesh	1989	China	1985
India	1986	Japan	1985
Nepal	1988	Singapore	1985
Sri Lanka	1986	Canada	1981
Thailand	1985	USA	1981
Pakistan	1987	Source: Park[xii]	

Introduction

In many western countries, such as Canada and US, HIV had initially been considered a disease primarily affecting intravenous drug users, blood product recipients, commercial sex workers (CSW's), and homosexuals. However, this has proven to be a misunderstanding of monumental proportion as women are now a growing segment of the infected population and can, in turn, pass the infection on to an unborn child[xiii]. In developing nations however, heterosexual activities accounts for 75% of transmission, both male and female. Women represent 40% of the estimated infected population[xiv]. The common cause is infidelity by the partner or the female being involved with the enormous commercial sex trade.

The projected infant and child deaths from AIDS may increase child mortality rates in developing countries by as much as 50%, thereby eradicatng the gains made in the recent past related to child survival rates. It is estimated that by the year 2000, 10 million children will be infected worldwide as a result of materno- foetal infection and blood product transmission.[xv]

Table 2. Global Trend of HIV Infection in 1999

Mode of Transmission	Percent
Sexual Intercourse	70-80%
Materno–Foetal	5-10%
Needle Sharing by Drug Users	5-10%
Blood Transfusion	3-5%
Accidental Needle Sticks by Health Workers	<0.01%

Source: UNAIDS[xvi]

1.2 Historical Approach

Epidemiologists and health researchers still debate the origin of the HIV. Theories abound that it is a botched invention targeting certain groups: Africans, homosexuals, drug users, etc.[xvii]. This conspiracy theory is likely untrue, and is only detrimental to the health of the PLWHA, as they feel victim of moral blame. A more likely explanation is that the virus existed undetected for many years in isolated villages of Africa. As a person can harbor the virus for many years before death and rural African villages have always had short life expectancies and high levels of infections that kill at an early age, the virus could have been infecting persons for a long time without notice. A further theory, and now somewhat accepted, is that the virus had sprung from infected monkeys to humans, as the viruses in the monkeys are genetically similar to that of human beings[xviii]. The virus is linked closely to the Simian Immunodeficiency Virus (SIV) seen in monkeys. It is not likely that other animal immunodeficiency lentiviruses such as EIV (equine), FIV(feline), and BIV (bovine) crossed into humans as these are species specific, unlike SIV[xix]. However, it must be noted that HIV-2 is more closely linked to SIV. It is speculated that the use of monkey blood in sexual stimulation, male blood for males, female blood for females, inoculated onto the pubic region in traditional superstitions provided the likely initial exposure. It is interesting to note that it was first in Cameroon that scientists discovered new strains of the virus, now reaching over thirty, that can often escape detection with standard ELISA testing. However, the belief that HIV began in Africa goes on to further stigmatize the situations there.

Retrospective investigations have been carried out on stored sera and other materials which were collected from different countries. A sample taken from Zaire, 1959, revealed HIV-1

Antibodies. AIDS was also the suspected cause of disease in a Norwegian family in the 1960's, and then death in 1976. However, the earliest case discovered is in the death of an English seaman from Manchester in 1959[xx]. There is no evidence that this man had been to Africa. One may, in fact, assume, as a result of the deaths, that HIV may have begun in the 1930's[xxi]. It is likely that many deaths went unrecognized.

■■

Chapter 2

DISEASE

2.1 Mode of Transmission

HIV is foremostly a sexually transmitted disease (STD). Any vaginal, anal, or oral sexual act can spread the virus. In developing nations, HIV is acquired mainly through heterosexual contact (male to female, female to male). Every act of unprotected intercourse with an HIV infected person exposes the uninfected partner to the risk of infection. The degree of risk is affected by several factors: the presence of an STD, the type of sexual act, the stage of illness of the infected partner, the use of sexual protection, etc. Studies indicate that a woman is twice as vulnerable to infection from a male as a male is from female[xxii] as a larger surface area is involved. The risk of infection in both sexes increases during female menstruation. Exposed adolescent girls and women approaching menopause are believed to be at greater risk than women between these life stages. In teenagers the cervix is thought to be a less efficient barrier to HIV than in the mature genital tract of adult women. The thinning of mucosa at menopause is also believed to lessen the protective barrier, whilst the production of mucus in the genital tract of adolescent girls and in menopausal women is not as rapid as in adult women, thus enhancing the chances of infection[xxiii].

Previous exposure to Sexually Transmitted Diseases correlates to increased incidence of HIV infection. An estimated 250 million people acquire STD's in a year[xxiv], it is, therefore, obvious why sexual intercourse has become the largest mode of transmission. An STD in either partner increases the likelihood of infection. If an STD, such as syphilis (a common STD in developing countries), causes ulceration in the genital or perineal region of the uninfected partner, it becomes easier for transmission to occur. An STD causes inflammation, therefore causing T- cells, monocytes and macrophages to concentrate in the genital area. This opening of the protective skin barrier allows transmission[xxv]. It should be noted here that despite hypothesis in the past, the link between syphilis and HIV infection is not *"hidden"*[1].

Table 3. Indian Trend of HIV infection in 1998

Mode of Transmission	Percent
Heterosexual Intercourse	73.6%
Homosexual Intercourse	0.8%
Blood Product Infusion/ needle sharing	10.2%
Blood Transfusion	6.6%
Others/ unavailable histories	8.8%
Total	100%
Source: UNAIDS[xxvi]	

Direct infection through contaminated blood may be a thing of the past in developed countries as blood is tested using the ELISA method, and factor VIII for haemophiliacs is heat treated[xxvii]. However, developing countries must see this mode of transmission as a realistic threat. The cost of screening blood often results in dishonest activities and so, the test is overlooked.

Contaminated blood is highly infective through transfusion and results in as much as 6.6% of infections in India[xxviii]. Other blood product infection depends on the amount of virions in the product. Infection through contaminated needles, syringes, or other skin piercing instruments is lower than other modes of transmission; however the use of shared needles among drug users is the cause of up to 10% of infections in India, as the exposure is repeated so often, possibly several times per day.

The materno- foetal transmission may also be considered largely a thing of the past in developed countries, as the early use of the drug Zididuvine (AZT) has reduced the transmission. However, as modern antiretroviral drugs are largely unavailable in developing nations, the materno foetal route accounts for up to 10% of the infection. The HIV may be passed from mother to child through the placenta, during delivery, or through breast feeding. As many as one third of the children of HIV+ve mothers become infected as a result of these modes of transmission. Often the children develop AIDS rapidly, and so, account for as high as 20% of AIDS cases.

2.2 Incubation Period

The fact, that this disease is relatively new poses the problem that the natural history and progression is not thoroughly understood. In developed countries the incubation period ranges from a few months to unlimited years. A small number of patients in Australia remain healthy despite having been infected for greater than seventeen years[xxix]. However, in developing countries, the duration is much shorter. The current average from time of exposure to time that AIDS begins is 4-6 years. Many factors can play a role in the expedient progression of developing nations infected individuals: lack of nutrition, poor medical advice, lack of sufficient medicaments, poor shelter, etc. The virus can often remain dormant in the system for years, and it is assumed that some infected individuals will never develop into AIDS stage. The "acute- mononucleosis like syndrome" several weeks after exposure is rarely seen in developing nations as acute fevers, malaise, arthralgias, and lymphadenopathy, and are usually treated by lay persons[xxx]. The "acute-mononucleosis like syndrome" correlates with antibody production, however, the antibodies will not inactivate the virus. Most persons will generally feel healthy from the time of infection until pathological changes occur, yet remain infectious to others. It should be well noted that during the asymptomatic periods, these HIV carriers should be considered individuals, not patients.

2.3 AIDS Related Complex (ARC) or Middle Stage HIV Infection:

The term ARC has been abandoned, as we now know that the ARC stage is a manifestation of middle stage HIV disease. Nonetheless, as ARC is universally understood, and still used in many settings, we shall give a description. The ARC is a constellation of chronic symptoms and signs manifested by HIV+ individuals who have not had the opportunistic infections or tumors, nor <200 CD4/uL, that define AIDS. They may exhibit clinical signs of unexplained diarrhoea, lasting more than one month, fatigue, malaise, fever, night sweats, oral and vaginal candidiasis, hairy leukoplakia, or generalized lymphadenopathy[xxxi]. A severe manifestation of ARC is the "wasting syndrome", also called "the slimming disease" in developing nations, usually considered if more than 15% of the total body weight is lost. Many patients with ARC will go on to develop AIDS.

2.4 Acquired Immuno Deficiency Syndrome (AIDS)

AIDS is characteristically defined in developed countries when the individual CD4+ count reaches <200/uL[xxxii]. However, perhaps a more consistent definition would be when the development of opportunistic infections and cancers becomes life threatening. The reasoning behind this change in definition is important for two reasons. Firstly, many patients in both developed and developing nations have been observed to be healthy whilst having CD4+ counts as low as 66/uL for extended periods of time. Similarly, in Canada, a patient was observed having a CD4+ count of 18/uL whilst remaining in resonally good health. Further to this, many patients in India have expired as a result of the disease whilst having relatively normal CD4+ counts. Secondly, as the majority of patients are aware that the AIDS stage is the final stage in the progression of the disease before death, it may preempt death to diagnose an apparently healthy individual to be in a fatal stage. As we shall later see, the psychological blow of the diagnosis can also affect the degree of health.

Table 4. Diseases Indicating AIDS, Without Laboratory Findings

Candidiasis of esophagus, trachea, bronchi, or lungs
Cryptococcosis outside the lungs
Cryptosporidial diarrhoea for >1 month
Cytomegalovirus infection exclusive of liver, spleen, or lymph nodes
Herpes simplex causing skin ulcers for > 1 month
Kaposi's sarcoma in patients < 60 years
Lymphoma of the brain in patients <60 years

Lymphoid interstitial pneumonitis

Disseminated mycobacterium avium complex infections

Pneumocystis carinii pneumonia

Progressive multifocal leukoencephalopathy or parvovirus encephalitis

Toxoplasmic encephalitis

Source: WHO[xxxiii]

Table 5. WHO Clinical Case Definition (for use when diagnostic tools are limited)

At least two major signs and one minor sign must be present to suggest infection

Major Signs:

    a) weight loss more than 10% of body weight

    b) fever for more than one month

    c) diarrhoea for more than one month

Minor signs:

    a) cough for more than one month

    b) generalized pruritic dermatitis

    c) recurrent herpes zoster or shingles

    d) oropharyngeal candidiasis or thrush

    e) chronic or aggressive ulcerative herpes simplex

    f) persistent generalized lymphadenopathy

Source: WHO[xxxiv]

In developed nations many of the infections mentioned in Table 4 may be observed in late stages of AIDS. However, in developing nations, the majority of the aforementioned diseases are not observed as the patients will often expire more rapidly as a result of tuberculosis infection[xxxv]. In countries where TB is endemic, many individuals are exposed during childhood. When the immune system is compromised, the infection recurs. In HIV patients, developing bacillemia will result in a higher proportion of tuberculous lesions extrapulmonary, making early diagnosis difficult. AIDS encephalopathy, or AIDS dementia, caused by the HIV crossing the "blood- brain barrier", is rarely seen in developing nations as the patient expires quickly.

Table 6. Opportunistic Infections

Protazoal:	Pneumocystis carinii
	Toxoplasma
	Cryptosporidium
Fungi:	Candida
	Cryptococcus
	Coccidioides
	Histoplasma
Viruses:	Cytomegalovirus
	Herpes simplex
	Epstein Barr virus
Bacteria:	Mycobacterium tuberculosis
	Atypical mycobacterium
	Legionella
	Source: Merck[xxxvi]

It should well be noted that many disease will cause a combination of the above mentioned symptoms, and so differentiation must be made from: tuberculosis, alcoholism, cancer, starvation, or leprosy.

2.5 Screening

At present the majority of developed countries offer free anonymous testing for antibodies to the HIV. Generally, these tests are paid for by the government social planning or health centers. HIV is unique in that anonymous testing is potentially available to all individuals[xxxvii], whereas all other laboratory tests for communicable diseases require a doctor's order. Blood tests are generally not required for travelling purposes, but may be necessary for immigration, marriage, birth planning, blood donors, or employment purposes; it is often in this manner that individuals are initially diagnosed.

In developing nations, blood testing is rarely available without a doctor's approval, and is rarely without cost. In India, the cost of an HIV test can be from R150($6 CAN.) to R2000($70 CAN.)[xxxviii], often out of reach for the inhabitants of poverty stricken areas. The test is rarely anonymous and may carry the immense social stigma resulting in social rejection and psychological consequences. Counselling, which is mandatory before testing, may often be overlooked or questionable. In the busier clinics, where testing is often done on-the-spot, the doctor or counsellors may not have the time to provide proper counselling and so, the patient will often leave in a state of panic or shock.

In rural areas of India, where medical help is poorly provided, the patients may remain undiagnosed to the point of death. It is rarely witnessed that patients will volunteer for testing. However, in larger cities, such as Mumbai, the individuals are often tested voluntarily or as a result of family planning routines, or job applications (consider the Middle East). An issue recently raised by Vinod Khanna, the popular film star turned right wing BJP member of parliament, that HIV testing should be made

Disease

mandatory and those testing positive should be made to wear badges[xxxix], is an example of how little understanding the government has.

2.6 Monitoring

Until recently, CD4+ cell count has been the standard marker for following the disease progression. Patients with a CD4+ count between 500-1300/uL were considered to be in normal health. CD4+ counts below 500/uL were considered to be in ARC stage and CD4+ below 200/uL were considered to be in AIDS, with <50/uL considered to be near death. However, the results of CD4+ monitoring have not always correlated to the patients general health as many patients with CD4+ <200/uL have had good states of health according to standard clinical observations. It has recently been the trend, in developed countries, to monitor more closely the viral load. It is now clear that the early stage of HIV infection that was previously assumed, when the CD4+ counts remain normal, may in fact, relate more to the constant battle between viral replication and lymphocyte proliferation.

In developing countries, viral load testing is unavailable; whilst CD4+ count testing is largely unavailable due to cost (approximately 700R, $25CAN)[xl]. Therefore, the clinical observations of experienced health care providers are the best indicators of disease progression.

■■

Chapter 3

EPIDEMIOLOGY

3.1 Epidemiological Features

Table 7. Epidemiological Model

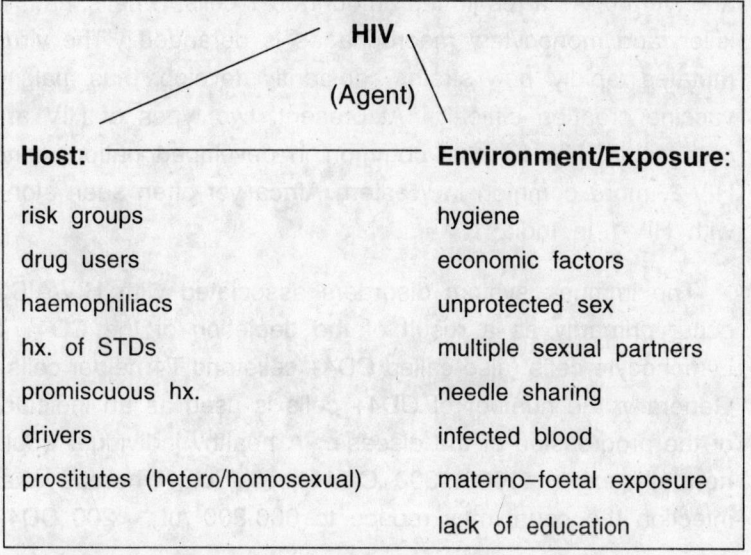

Host:

risk groups
drug users
haemophiliacs
hx. of STDs
promiscuous hx.
drivers
prostitutes (hetero/homosexual)

Environment/Exposure:

hygiene
economic factors
unprotected sex
multiple sexual partners
needle sharing
infected blood
materno–foetal exposure
lack of education

3.2 Agent

When the virus was first identified it was called "lymphadenopathy Associated Virus" (LAV) by the French team of scientists claiming its discovery, and "Human T- cell Lymphotropic Virus III"(HTLV III) by the American joint team also claiming discovery, and also called AIDS associated Retrovirus (ARV)[xli]. It was not until May 1986 that the universal name Human Immunodeficiency Virus (HIV) was decided upon. The tiny virus (1/10'000th of a millimetre in diameter) is in a protein capsule containing RNA and enzymes. As with all retroviruses, an enzyme called reverse transcriptase that converts viral RNA into proviral DNA copy that becomes integrated into the host cell DNA. These integrated proviruses are duplicated with normal cellular genes during each cell division. The HIV replicates mainly in the T4 lymphocytes, upsetting T4 helper cell genesis. The virus has the ability to cross the blood- brain barrier and can affect the microglial cells of the brain. HIV greatly affects the dendritic cells of the skin and lymph. As a result, the amount of T cells, B cells, natural killer, and monocytes/ macrophages is deranged. The virus mutates rapidly, new strains constantly develop, thus making vaccine creation difficult. At present, two types of HIV are recognized, HIV-1, most common in developed nations, and HIV-2, more common in Western Africa yet often seen along with HIV-1 in India[xli].

The immune system disorders associated with HIV/AIDS occur primarily as a result of the depletion of the CD4+ T Lymphocyte cells (also called CD4+ cells and T4 helper cells). Generally, the number of CD4+ cells is used as an indicator of the progression of the disease. A healthy individual would normally exhibit 1000-1300 CD4+ cells /uL, whereas after infection the count may reduce to 600-800 /uL, <200 CD4+

Table 8. Epidemiological factors

PERIOD OF PRE-PATHOGENESIS

HIV *(agent)*

RISK GROUPS *(host)*   *(environment)*
- political, economic factors
- education
- availability of information, testing
- condoms, IV needles

WEIGHT<

PERIOD OF PATHOGENESIS

                  DEATH

          AIDS (cancers, opp. infections, retinitis)

    MALAISE, OPPORTUNISTIC INFECTIONS, CD4<

  ARC
(GPL, THRUSH FEVER, DIARRHOEA,

CD4 COUNTS<

HIV
LATENT PERIOD
(asymptomatic)

AGENT BECOMES ESTABLISHED AND MULTIPLIES

Continue

LEVELS of PREVENTION	PRIMARY PREVENTION	SECONDARY PREVENTION	TERTIARY PREVENTION
Modes of Intervention:	Health Promotion:	Diagnosis	Disability limitations:
- public education-safe sex	Treatment with:		- financial support
- professional education	-safe blood transfusions	- allopathy	- familial empowerment
- community attitudes	-decreasing needle sharing	- homoeopathy	- community " "
	-education	- counselling	- spiritual counselling
			- social networks

Epidemiology 21

/uL is considered end stage HIV, or AIDS[xliii]. These numbers however, are questionable.

The reservoir of infection in the case of HIV is human. The infected individuals will remain so for life long, at present. Since HIV infected individuals may not develop symptoms for several years, they may be considered infectious from the inception of infection. It is interesting to note that individuals are considered more infectious during the very early stages, the "window period" before antibody production has mounted a defense; and again later as the disease reaches an advanced stage as the immune system is severely compromised.

3.3 Host

Most HIV infections have occurred among sexually active adults between the age of 20-49 yrs. This group represents the most sexually active, as well as leading high risk lifestyles. However, the number of children and elderly being infected is growing at an alarming rate. The majority of infections in developing nations are caused by heterosexual activities; heterosexual activities with multiple partners, commercial sex workers, and anal intercourse increases the likelihood of transmission.

Chapter 4

ENVIRONMENT

4.1 HIV in India

The WHO recent estimates of reported HIV in India exceeds the number of 2,000000, and current Indian estimates around 10,000,000[xliv]. We shall shortly explain why the latter number more correctly represents the actual amount of HIV+ individuals. India offers little hope for individuals diagnosed as having the HIV, as successful anti–retroviral drugs are largely unaffordable[xlv]. As the current rate of infection soars in India, it is necessary to examine different therapies that may provide some relief, or hope, to the People Living With HIV and AIDS (**PLWHA**). Many therapies claim to be beneficial or effective in the treatment of HIV and so closer examination has been necessary.

The first confirmed reports of HIV infection in India came in April 1986, when six commercial sex workers in Tamil Nadu were found positive for HIV antibodies[xlvi]. Several studies have subsequently been initiated for prevalence measurement. However, the reported prevalence of infection represents only a fraction of actual morbidity. The spread of HIV in India is most often due to unprotected heterosexual activities (homosexual activities are not a major factor as homosexuality is shunned and often repressed), usually with Commercial Sex Workers (CSWs). Heterosexual sex accounts for close to 80% of infection in India[xlvii]. Prior infection with other STD's increases the likelihood of HIV infection. The initial spread of HIV was blamed on prostitutes in urban areas, related to immigration. It was estimated that four to five years ago there were 160,000 prostitutes working in Bombay, presently there are an estimated 70,000, as a result of AIDS[xlviii]. Many medical personnel in India have blamed truck drivers for the quick spread of HIV in the late eighties and early nineties due to the accepted use of prostitutes at truck-stops for long journeys; the drivers later return to their families and infect them[xlix]. This is a common situation seen in the clinics as young children are often left parentless and forced to live on the streets; they become a part of the epidemic's cycle (See photo 1.5). A present estimate by the Health Action Information Network (HAIN) has put the percentage of drivers infected by HIV at 25%[l]. The prevalence of HIV infection among long route drivers is highest. Alarming reports are now coming from the national highway 8, between Jaipur and Bombay. Studies done in Manipur have shown a high prevalence of STD and HIV at places where trucks traditionally halt[li]. The truckers explain that the prevalence of unsafe, risky sexual practices amongst them, which includes unprotected sex with commercial sex workers, men, and *hijras* (hermaphrodites and eunuchs), is but an outcome and index of their loneliness; performed without thinking, under the influence of *afeem* (opium) and alcohol. They say that without these indulgences, the life on the road is harder to bear[lii]. (See case example #1) A victim of the moral blame are the *hijras* (hermaphrodites or eunuchs, see photo # 1.3), already shunned by society due to their differences, these are blamed as the initial and constant spread of the disease due to the number working as cheap prostitutes at truck stops[liii]. While the major route of infection is by heterosexual promiscuity, the prevalence of disease is high in intravenous drug users who share syringes and needles. A mention should be made of Manipur. The studies conducted by the Field Practice Unit of Surveillance Center for HIV Infection at Imphal, have shown that incidence in Manipur is high as a result of easily obtainable injectable heroin. The first sero- positive case in Manipur was detected in 1989, yet within three years, 1600 cases were reported. There are 15'000 to 20'000 drug users in the state, out of a total population of 1.8 million[liv].

Both HIV-1 and HIV-2 are present in India, however HIV-1 is predominantly the infectious agent in a large number of cases. It has previously been theorized by some in the medical community that infection by HIV- 2, the less severe strain, may prevent infection by HIV-1. However, as is the case in many of the patients examined, both HIV-1 & 2 can frequently infect the same individual. It must be noted that many of the patients in Gujarat had been infected through blood transfusion. It has not been until 1994 that screening blood for any diseases became common in government hospitals[lv]. However, as government hospitals are not respected by most individuals, alternate hospitals and clinics are normally used for common ailments. These private hospitals purchase their blood from blood banks. The blood banks test blood at 150Rs ($6CAN) per pint and will in turn sell the blood for 900Rs ($32CAN) per pint[lvi]. This is not feasible for most of the patients and so they will opt for untested blood; particularly those who are exceptionally poor or uneducated. Untested blood is of major concern as it is sheer ignorance of the laboratory personnel to allow the blood to be dispensed untested (See case example #2).

The vast majority of HIV patients were diagnosed as a result of suspicion by the attending physician, particularly as the

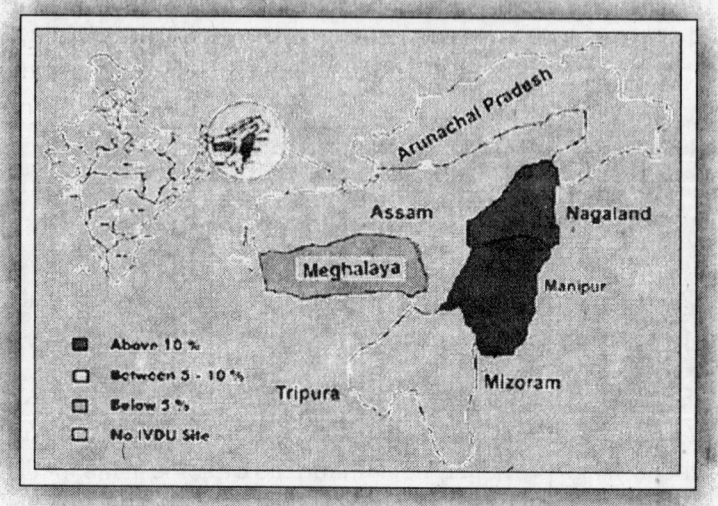

Figure 1.1 : Prevalence of IV Drug Users in North Eastern India

patient presents with common symptoms that are not responding to typical therapies; such as TB or fevers. Often patients in the hospital for seemingly common ailments will be observed with persistent generalized lymphadenopathy, oral thrush and ulcers, recurrence of herpes zoster, persistent diarrhoea, or rapid loss of weight; AIDS related complex has begun and the immune system is compromised. At this time the patients will be recommended an HIV test, which they must pay for; ranging in price from 150Rs to 2000Rs. It is unfortunate, but the vast majority of patients will not go for the test either due to moral concern or financial hardship, and will therefore, not be diagnosed at an early stage. Considering that there is no benefit to the patient to be aware of his status, as they will not receive any different treatment than their symptomatic allopathic treatment, it is not surprising that the patients are often unwilling to go for expensive testing. It is, therefore, reasonable to suggest, that the majority of infected individuals are unaware, and that the number of occurrence far exceeds that noted by the WHO.

Once the patient has been diagnosed as HIV+ a system of counselling is developed. No allopathic treatment is prescribed as the cost is generally not possible for the patient. The antiretroviral drug Zydovidine costs a monthly 30'000Rs[lvii]; impossible for the average HIV+ individual who earns a monthly 1000Rs ($35 CAN)[lviii]. The patients are informed to no longer put other individuals at risk through sexual activities and blood donations. The patients are normally advised to inculcate hygienic habits and promote regular bathing. A proteinous diet is normally recommended, with avoidance of meat and other foods that are difficult to digest. Addictions are recommended to cease, such as coffee and tea intake, as well as alcohol, afeem, cigarettes, chewing tobacco and pan (a tobacco related product). The patients will receive counselling and allopathic support ranging from biweekly in asymptomatic cases to everyday in later stages of AIDS. There are, however, no staff in the area of Anand (Gujarat State), who are entirely devoted to HIV treatment with patients. Unfortunately, it is often the case that the patients do not follow the advice of their health workers, and will simply carry on with their regular life; putting themselves and others at risk.

Rural Indian health education is poor and so, one will often find the compliance rate of the patients to be inconsistent. Another difficulty in rural areas is the misunderstanding of the disease and treatment. The disease is often seen as a punishment. One example of this; a patient from a poor background, had borrowed and spent 60'000Rs on alternative treatments such as ayurveda and, unfortunately, witchcraft. The witch doctor consumed a large amount of the money and informed the patient that the reason for the infection was evil spirits, that he must be cleansed of his evil acts. Not surprisingly, a patient under this type of moral attack will not thrive and the patient expired whilst this research was being conducted[lix].

Suicide is an unfortunate sequelae to this disease, related to the guilt, shame, and misunderstanding of their situation. Whilst undertaking this study, one female patient committed suicide, and one male patient, aged 65, attempted suicide. The older patient later refused food, water, or medications, even though he was asymptomatic. Counselling is, of course, a necessary therapy, particularly when families are not present or not accepting; however, the common situation of lack of funding and staff exists.

Further stigma is often created by the medical community and public health educators; for example, in 1987 the Indian Council for Medical Research issued guidelines that the dead body of a person with HIV needs to be sprinkled with Sodium Hypochlorate (bleach) and be double wrapped in polyethylene or plastic before being handed over to relatives. Although this guideline was later withdrawn, its guidelines are still being meticulously followed by many healthcare institutions[lx]. It thus forms the basis of the ultimate discrimination of people living and dying with HIV, even in death. A conversation with Dr. J. Shah, a prominent paediatric surgeon in Vadodara resulted in his explanation as to not operating on a 7 day old child "why should I touch him, he has AIDS, he is as good as dead[lxi]", a common misconception according to Dr. Pankaj Dave, a leading homoeopath in the same town[lxii]. Perhaps the misconception can be further linked to the public health educational posters displaying slogans such as "AIDS is DEATH"[lxiii].

Often the patients will undergo a period of shock related to the diagnosis. The patients are aware that there is no cure for AIDS and expect imminent death. The patients are most often afraid of the stigma of the disease by the Indian culture, who victimize the patient. It is often the case that the family will blame the patient and illtreat him; there was one patient who was kept outside by her family. There is no social support system in India for the sick, and so often hospitals do not seek long term treatment of the chronically ill, as the cost is too high. Due to the lack of social assistance, the patient's families are put at risk sperially if the patient has been the breadwinner. It is the tradition in India for the wife to care for the dying husband, leaving the obvious problem once the husband has deceased and the wife becomes ill. It is an unfortunate fact that unless the parents of the husband or wife are alive and accepting, that the wife may die alone. (See case example #2)

As most patients are diagnosed whilst having HIV related infections or AIDS, the average length of time for a patient in India to survive after diagnosis is one to three years[lxiv]. The most common morbific agent related to death is tuberculosis. The presence of HIV infection greatly increases the chances that bacillemia will accompany what otherwise would be simply self limiting primary TB. As a result, a large proportion of tuberculous lesions in HIV infected individuals are extrapulmonary[xlv]; with the opportunistic TB infection reaching the Waldeyer ring, lymph nodes, abdominal organs, bones, and joints. Tuberculosis and other respiratory ailments more often result in death before the characteristic symptoms of AIDS develop: Kaposi's sarcoma, dementia, blindness, paralysis. Pneumocystis carinii pneumonia (PCP) is not often diagnosed in India; more commonly, it is diagnosed as pneumonia. It is the intention, and encouraged by the reasonable hospitals that the patients be allowed to die at home with their family, if accepted, to allow them to die with dignity. It is unfortunate, but due to a lack of staff, the patients will often pass away without any medical staff being aware.

There are many reasons that the average length of time between infection with HIV and death is much shorter in India than in developed countries. The obvious lack of hygiene and nutrition is certainly a factor, as disease thrives in the warm climate and fatal diseases are numerous (See Photo 1.2, 1.4, 1.5 & 1.6); note that TB and malaria are considered endemic to most northern regions. The obvious lack of antiviral drugs certainly accounts for the rapid decline in the health of the patients. But let us also take into consideration the commonplace procedure of self prescribing or layman prescribing in most ailments. Prescriptions are generally not required at pharmacies and antibiotics, anti- malarial, and anti-psychotic drugs are used sporadically by the majority of individuals. The patient generally does not finish a course of antibiotics and returns the unused portions to the pharmacy for a refund[lxvi]. This process increases the likelihood of opportunistic infections and superinfections. It must be noted that a large proportion of the medical personnel practicing as allopaths may, in fact, not have finished allopathic medical college[lxvii]. A good example of medical ignorance related to HIV is at the Karnataka Institute of Medical Sciences where the ELISA testing kits had been lying around unused for the last year as a result of "lack of expertise", the first HIV testing at the hospital began on November 27, 1999[lxviii]. Health in India is most often compromised due to lack of education. Lack of education in the case of HIV, results in massive amounts of unsafe sex with high risk individuals (See case example #4), unsafe blood transfusions, and poor hygiene. The misinformation is a substantial threat to the health of the population, for example, on the 1st of December 1999, Dr. S. Subramanya of the Karnataka State AIDS prevention Society released a media statement that *"the new drug available, AZT, stops the infection inutero. This means that an HIV+ couple can now have children without fear"*, the article goes on to say misinform that AZT is widely available[lxix]. It has been argued by many NGO's that the government is doing too little, too late. It is then reassuring when the Union Health Minister, Mr. Shanaranand went on record saying "AIDS is not a problem in India and moreover, there is a cure for AIDS in Belgaum, my home constituency".[lxx]

4.2 Opportunistic Infections

The first case of AIDS in India was reported in 1986. Subsequently, a surveillance system was developed in 1987. The data from this surveillance activity suggests that the HIV infection has now spread to the general population and to all parts of the country, except Arunachal Pradesh in North-eastern India. With the changing scenario of the AIDS epidemic, a host of opportunistic infections add to the present endemic state of some already existing infections like tuberculosis. This report analyses the AIDS cases in India, reported to the National AIDS Control Organization over the years between 1986 to 1997. A total of 3,551 AIDS cases had been reported till 31st May 1997. Tuberculosis (pulmonary and extrapulmonary) is the major opportunistic infection affecting 62% of the cases followed by candidiasis seen in 57% of the patients. In 1997, of the 390 AIDS cases analysed, tuberculosis (pulmonary and extrapulmonary) accounted for 56.5% of the total cases whereas candidiasis was seen in 61% of the cases. An increasing trend was observed with tuberculosis from 58% in 1986-1992 to 68.5% in 1995. No trend could be established in the case of candidiasis, though, a high prevalence of 66% was seen in the cases between 1986 and 1992. An increase was also observed in cases of PCP, cerebral toxoplasmosis and Kaposi sarcoma. In the AIDS cases, chronic diarrhea (76%), weight loss (87%) and fever (85%) appeared to be the major presenting symptoms. But, of the 390 AIDS cases reported in 1997, only 47% of them were suffering from chronic diarrhea. With increase in the number of AIDS cases, India is burdened with a dual epidemic of HIV/AIDS and tuberculosis. The National AIDS Control Organization in India, is involved in training clinicians and laboratory personnel in the diagnosis and management of the AIDS cases. With better diagnosis of the opportunistic infections, especially diarrhea, in AIDS patients, a better picture will emerge regarding the opportunistic infections which would help clinicians and health planners to tackle the AIDS epidemic in a more effective manner.[lxxi]

4.3 Indian AIDS History

- April 1986: First cluster (10) prostitutes of HIV seropositives detected in Chennai, Tamil Nadu.
- May 1986: First AIDS patient detected in Bombay (recipient of unscreened blood transfusion from USA).
- December 1986: 1st seropositive male detected at STD clinic in Tamil Nadu.
- July 1987: 1st seropositive blood donor detected in Vellore, Tamil Nadu.
- July 1987: 1st spouse to spouse transmission detected (abovementioned donor's wife).
- October 1987: 1st detection of a seropositive infant (born to above-mentioned couple).
- April 1988: 1st indigenous case of AIDS in an Indian.

- January 1989: Evidence of HIV in indigenously produced blood products.
- May 1989: Central Council for Research in Homoeopathy (CCRH) begins pilot research project of 129 HIV carriers.
- July 1989: Government notification for mandatory blood screening of donated blood.
- January 1990: Recognition of HIV+ clusters in IV drug users.
- November 1992: CCRH releases results of homoeopathic drug trials.
- July 1992: Constitution of the National AIDS control Organizations at state levels.
- October 1992: Establishment of the National AIDS Research Institute, Pune, by Indian Council for Medical Research (ICMR)
- July 1992: Human Intracisternal Retrovirus reported.
- August 1995: CCRH release study *Homoeopathic Drugs as Immunomodulators*.
- January 1996: Professional blood donors outlawed.
- July 1998: Dr. K.M. Pavri from the National Institute of Virology (NIV) in Pune had reported particles of a retrovirus in an asymptomatic pregnant prostitute (one of the first ten discovered in Tamil Nadu in 1986). This is termed Idiopathic CD4+ T lymphocytopaenia.

4.4 Case Example #1

35 year old Mr. S. had been a patient of Dr. Kaushal Jain for several years. Mr. S. was a truck driver, living in Baroda, yet commuting to and from Ahmedabad and Bombay frequently on highway 8, a distance of 511kms. Dr. Jain had warned Mr. S in the past about the perils of frequenting the truck stop

sex workers, particularly since he was a husband and father. Dr. Jain recommended that if he felt that commercial sex was necessary, then a condom was absolutely necessary as a precaution for HIV and other STD's. Over the years Mr. S had been infected with gonorrhoea several times, yet always received standard allopathic treatment, with success. During the last gonorrheal infection Dr. Jain recommended that as a precaution he should volunteer for an HIV test. The results were positive, and Dr. Jain had to deliver the shocking news. Since that period, the patient is under the homoeopathic treatment of Dr. Jain. Mr. S. remains in health.

4.5 Case Example #2

Four years ago Mr.A. was in a motor vehicle accident resulting in a severe head injury. Mr.A. was treated at a private hospital in Anand, Gujarat, and received minor surgery and a blood transfusion. Mr. A., originally from Maharashtra, had come with his family several years before to Gujarat in an effort to escape the poverty of his home town; he bagan to work selling vegetables in the Anand market. Three years after the accident Mr.A. began to suffer from prolonged fevers and diarrhoea, and was attended to by the Emery Hospital staff. Dr. S. Christian, the attending physician, recommended an HIV test, however the cost (150Rs) was too much for the family and hence the test was delayed. Subsequently, the hospital provided the test free of charge and the results confirmed that Mr.A. was HIV+. Unfortunately, Mr.A. was never to recover from his illness and died on Christmas day 1998, a day when the hospital was closed, and so no medical attention was made available due to cost. During several visits to Mr. A.'s family of a wife and four small children, it was easily observable that their grief was very much present. Since the time of the diagnosis, the wife has also tested positive for HIV. There is not much hope for the family as they are presently surviving on the 500Rs ($17 CAN) per month that she is able to earn by cleaning houses. The widow and mother can not be expected to live for long as she is in a continuous state of grief and suffers from hunger. This will be another example of how the ignorance of some medical personnel has resulted in the devastation of entire families.

4.6 Case Example #3

Young Priti is five years old. She has just began her 1st standard at the local primary school. Both the Priti's parents died over the last three years as a result of their HIV status. Priti received the infection during birth when no-one was aware of their HIV status. She is presently taken care of by her ailing grandmother, but one cannot tell how long that will last. See attached photo.

4.7 Case Example #4

One patient at the hospital, the husband of patient X1-98, divorced his wife after discovering that she was a prostitute. He subsequently banished her from the house and town. His HIV+ status was only realized as a result of the wife's infection. Despite receiving counselling and educational materials, including condoms, the man remarried within three weeks without telling the new wife of his condition, and began to have unprotected sex. By the time that this was realized by the field team, several weeks had passed. His new wife has since tested positive for the virus. Both husband and wife have inquired if the wife can have her tubal ligotomy reversed, as they now wish to have children.

4.8 Case Example #5

The field team at the Emery hospital regularly visited Mr. and Mrs. Patel, residing in an extremely poor village approximately 2km. from Anand. The husband had contracted HIV from visits to a local CSW. The fact that the marital sexual relations were waning has, in fact, saved the wife from infection, as she has tested negative. Neither husband nor wife have ever attended formal education. On the fourth visit since diagnosis the husband was absent, he had returned to work. The wife informed us that her brother-in-law is a Hindu priest, and has informed the couple that the infection is not real. The couple took the advice of the priest and had an ox slaughtered in sacrifice to the God Maribhai, as well as payed 500Rs ($17CAN) to the priest. Whilst this is obviously not a cure, the patient's spiritual faith may work to some degree in improving the quality of life.

Chapter 5

DEMOGRAPHICS

5.1 Demographics

Whilst this disease certainly knows no boundaries of age, sex, religion, or economics, perhaps some groups may rightfully be labeled *high risk*. Indian literacy rates may be blamed for the lack of sex education that would normally be achieved in school!. However, sex education at the school level often lacks in duty, in an effort to promote traditional morals.

5.2 Migration and Employment

Bombay is said to have the largest amount of HIV+ people of any urban community in South East Asia[lxxii]. This is likely due to the large number of migrants from rural areas, in search of a better future[lxxiii]. The literacy rate amongst the migrants is shockingly low, and so the public health education is without effect. Another major reason is the presence of legalized commercial sex districts. Whilst the legalized commercial sex districts of developed countries, such as Holland, Germany, or Australia, enforce regular HIV testing of the people working there, little, if any rules apply in developing countries.

Commercial Sex Workers (CSW's) are in the highest risk groups, particularly in urban areas. The young people are often from rural backgrounds with little formal education, many come from poorer countries such as Bangladesh or Nepal (See photo 2.3). The legalized Commercial Sex Districts or "Red Light Districts" are filled with young girls with little chance of escape. Often the girls have been brought to Mumbai with promises of entering the film business, or of other dream jobs; nonetheless, resulting in horrific acts, and inevitable death. According to the Indian Health Organization (IHO), 60% of the 70'000 Mumbai Commercial Sex Workers (CSW) are said to be infected[lxxiv]. The studies reveal that on average a CSW will have three sexual contacts in a night. Thus, on any given night 132'000 sexual contacts that could result in HIV infection occur. Given that due to public health education, up to 70% of the sexual contacts may use protection, there is still a risk of almost 40'000 infections occurring. The CSW's will often request the client to use a condom, however, often the client will refuse. If the client reports that the CSW will not provide to the Madame, the CSW runs the risk of being homeless. Sexual intercourse in these areas costs as little as 5Rs (15 cents CAN). There is little hope for the young women, as the disease will inevitably infect them. There are several NGO's that can provide bare medical help, and in emergency, temporary shelter.

Table 9 : Rising Incidence of HIV in Commercial Sex Workers, 1987-1997, Mumbai

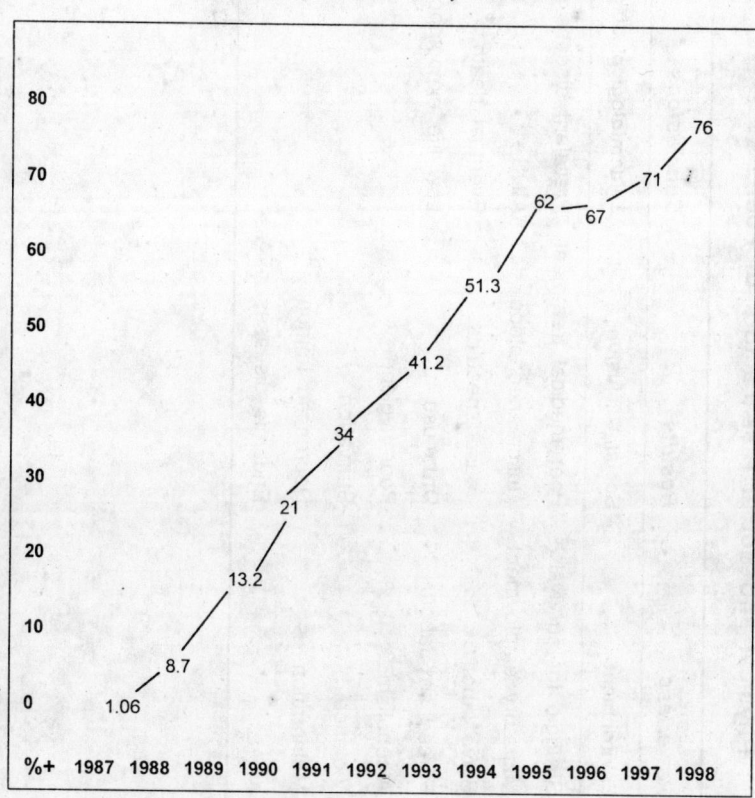

Source: Dr. G Bhave, AIDS Surveillance Centre, KEM Hospital, Mumbai

Table 10 : Physical and Social Risk Factors of Poor

Social Status	Powerless	Results	Conclusions
Predisposing Factors	Environment	Social Occlusion	Epidemiological diagnosis
Poverty	Struggle for survival	Poor medical treatment	Prevalent disease
Caste	Migratory employment	-unscreened blood	AIDS
Chronic illness	Slave labor	-reused needles	Eventual death
Lack of political power	Forced sex labour	Drug use	Low life expectancy
Lack of resources	Alcoholism	Poor hygiene	
Lack of education	Violence	Starvation	
Lack of healthcare	Malnutrition	Decreased Immunity	
Female		Endemic diseases	

Demographics 41

5.3 Women

What is of particular concern in this country is that women have become far more vulnerable to the virus than before, whether as a result of forced sex work or at the hands of an unfaithful spouse. The facts of increased numbers of infection among women are startling, though agencies and governments have not attempted efforts in this vein. AIDS is still viewed as predominantly a man's disease, since it is presumed that only men have sexual freedom. In India, the prevalence of infection in women is still only four to one, men to women, but quickly growing. Women are biologically at a greater risk and in addition face a number of social factors which contribute to making them more vulnerable to HIV and a quicker progression to AIDS. Across the social spectrum, they face limited access to health care and information regarding the functioning of their bodies. Most Indian women suffer from anemia as a result of which they require more blood transfusions than men, therefore increasing the likelihood of infection[lxxv]. As women lack employment opportunities and are often deprived of their right to inheritance and land, they are unable to negotiate social contracts despite being at risk. For example, most women lack the ability to deny conjugal rights to their husband, even if he has been unfaithful. A further example may be that rape is so often not reported, as the woman can be blamed.

A study by the Tata Institute of social Sciences, Mumbai, documented several traumatic cases suffered by women. Kanti, a 28 year old positive woman explained " my husband explained about AIDS to me but continued to have relations with me. I asked if it was okay and he said there was no problem, what could I do?"[lxxvii]. This is often seen more extremely in cases where HIV+ mothers suffer the trauma of being taken away from their children. Sindhu, a 32 year old HIV+ mother says

Table 11 : Rising Incidence of HIV in Women Attending Antenatal Clinics 1990- 1997, Mumbai

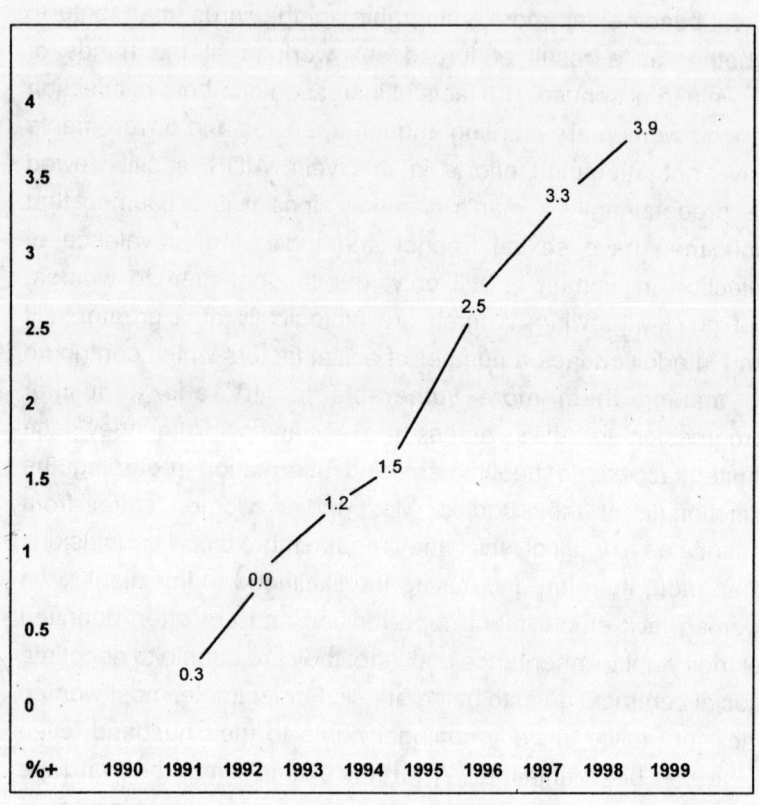

Source: Dr. G. Bhave, AIDS surveillance Centre, KEM hospital, Mumbai

" they (in-laws) keep my children with them. They let me visit, but do not allow me to come close to them. I still pay for the children's things. I have to be satisfied with this arrangement." In conservative societies, as is the case in India, women seeking information about HIV/AIDS may be considered indecent. Myths and superstitions heighten the risk to women. Men seek out

Demographics 43

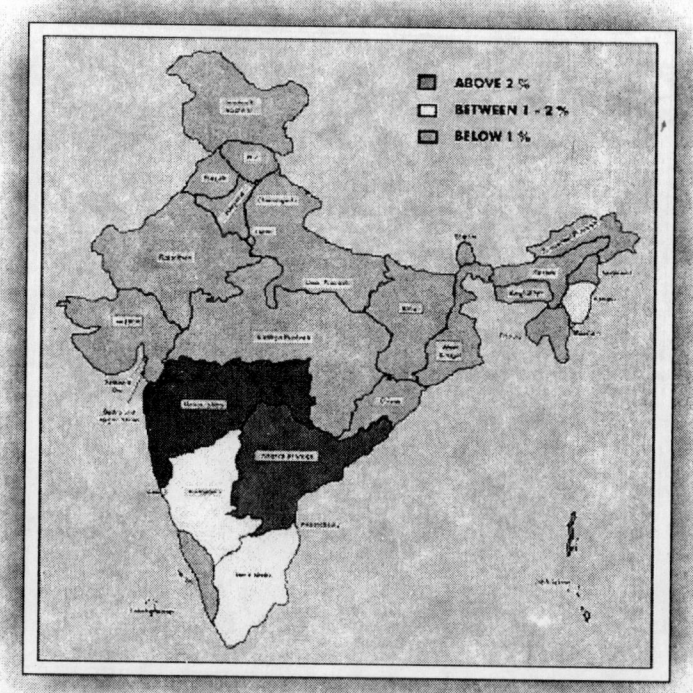

Figure 1.2 : Rising Incidence of Women Attending Clinics, 1998, National

Source : NACO[lxxvi]

ever younger female partners in the belief that they are less likely to contract any disease. In many parts of India and the world, the myth still exists that sex with a virgin actually cures men of various STD's.

5.4 Ethics

The shame that exists with this disease brings into question the notion of confidentiality. Of course, the patient's privacy

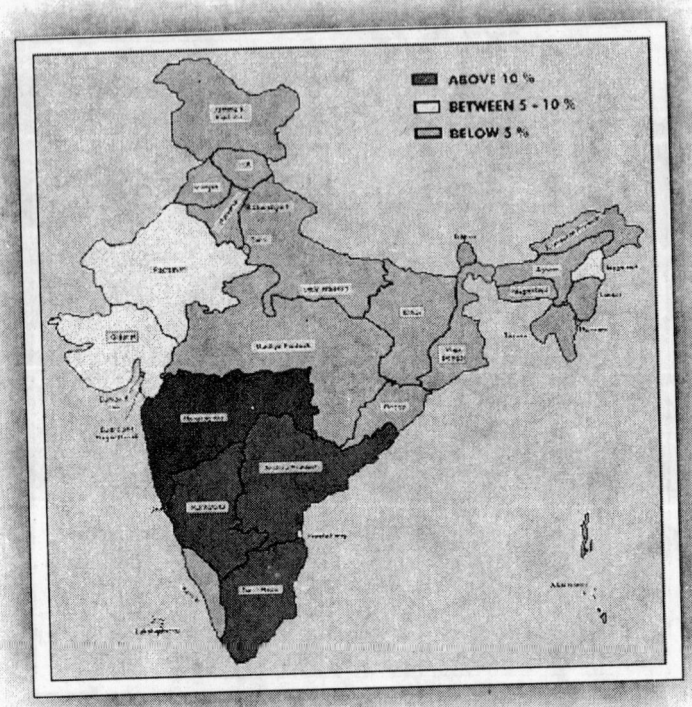

Figure 1.3 : STD Clinic Attendees, 1998, National
Source : NACO[lxxix]

must be secured; however, the ethic of doing no harm is more important to the public. If the patient refuses to divulge to his/ her spouse of his/ her positive status, should the doctor do so, thus breaking confidentiality? It is the primary calling of the physician to prevent sickness. Let us examine cases where the doctor could prevent further infections.

Case i. Case of HIV+ve prostitute married to HIV+ve man, After his discovery that she worked as a prostitute he threw her out of the house and remarried within two weeks, thus infecting the new spouse.

Case ii. HIV+ve man, diagnosed by doctor J.K., is set to be married by arranged marriage in summer. Dr. J.K. demands that the patient call off the marriage, threatening that if he does not, he will inform the bride.

The patient has rights but also obligations to do no harm themselves. Section 269 of the Indian Penal Code notes a provision for negligent act likely to cause infection of disease dangerous to life. This section was provided during the Raj to prevent the spread of plague, cholera, etc. Section 270 reads "malignant act likely to spread infection of disease dangerous to life with imprisonment of up to 2 years or fine, or both"[lxxviii]

Chapter 6

INFORMATION, EDUCATION, COMMUNICATION, COMPASSION.

6.1 Group I, Professional (Page-48)

6.2 Group II, General Population (Page-49)

6.3 Group III, Vulnerable Groups (Page-50)

6.4 Group IV, High Risk Groups (Page-51)

6.5 Group V, HIV+ and AIDS patients (Page-52)

Table : Group I, Professional

Type	Objectives	Initiative	Group Training	Method
Medical profession	Develop helping and positive attitude about patients.	Compassion for patients	NGO's	School visits
Healers		Understand psychosocial health	Medical faculties	Home visits
Nurses	Ensure equal rights of patients- destroy bias	Family planning education -sex education	Hospital Admin.	Up to date manuals for therapeutics
Lab. techs.	Ensure psychoneuroimmunity -counselling	Networks- specialists	Blood banks	Orientation meetings
Social Workers	Respect each others abilities in HIV -destroy bias	Networks- social groups	University/Colleges	Networks
Teachers	Research- between clinics - communication	Necessity for action	Schools	
Youth Leaders	Emergency networks	Emergency settings	Churches	
Religious Leaders	Discussion of sex matters -sex education	Understand confidentiality		
	Dispel myths	Hygiene in work and play		
		Common sense precautions -clinical settings -i.e. blood transfusions		
		Pre and post test counselling		
		Understand- history of disease - global implications -progress -social factors		
		Recognize clinical manifestations		
		Awareness of familial environment -behaviours		
		Collect funding		
		Voluntary work		
		Acknowledge poverty as a factor		

Table : Group II, General Population

Type of Group	Objectives	Initiative	Training	Method
Young men	Full knowledge of STD's, AIDS, its spread, prevention, and manifestations	Use of condoms	Teachers	Meetings
Young women	Destroy social stigma of AIDS	Dangers of -drugs -unsafe sex -prostitutes -promiscuity	Religious leaders	Mass media- TV -papers
Parent groups	Sexual education- safe sex - acknowledge sexuality		Youth groups	-booklets
			Doctors	-posters
	Avoid high risk situations	Develop volunteer groups	Counseling agencies	-leaflets
		Accepting HIV+ people	Social clubs	-drama
	Explain medical approaches and shortcomings	Collect funding	Gov't agencies	-pop music
			Village elders	Libraries

Table : Group III, Vulnerable Groups

Type of Group	Objectives	Initiative	Training	Method
Young adults	Education and understanding of STD's and AIDS	Dispel fears	Teachers	Meetings- group
Engaged couples	Sex education- puberty	Accept responsibility of actions	Youth groups	- 1 to 1
Unemployed	-reproduction	Moral understanding	Social workers	Educational films
Alcoholics	-condoms	Dangers of casual affairs	Religious groups	Role play/ drama
Women of child bearing age	-cause and spread of HIV	→sp. travelling	NGO's	Group discussion
Pregnant and lactating mothers	Acceptance of peers	What does not cause HIV	Employment agencies	Media
Labourers	Demand use of sterile needles -screened blood		Employers	Libraries
Uneducated	Avoid tattoos, drugs, prostitutes		Parents	
Homosexuals	Discussion in households		Women's groups	
	Information on free & confidential counselling and testing		Prostitute groups	
	Information on free medical treatment		Doctors	
	Dispel myths			
	Encourage acceptance of HIV+			

Table : Group IV, High Risk Groups

Type of Group	Objectives	Initiative	Training	Method
Prostitutes	Understand spread and prevention of STD's	Change of behaviour	NGO's	1-1 counsel
-Clients		Knowledge of STD's	Govt. hospitals	Audio/ visual aids
Patients w/ history of STD's	Use of safe sex -demand condoms	Use of condoms	Private clinics	Demonstrate condom Lectures
Promiscuous-hetero-	Sexual education	Responsibility towards spouse	Workplace-unions -health dept.	Free condoms
-bi-	Increase hygiene- oral -genitourinary	Pre & post-test counselling	Prostitutes organizations	-IV syringes
-homo-sexuals	-menstrual	Dispel fears	STD clinics	Musical groups
IV drug users	Regular testing		Volunteer groups	
Jail inmates	Avoid promiscuity		Spouse/ family	
Haemophiliacs	Communication w/ local help groups			
Thallasemics				
CRF patients				
Sailors	Disposal of syringes, condoms, soiled wastes			
Truck drivers	Education on living w/ HIV			
Professional blood donors	Dispel myths Acceptance of HIV+ people			

Table : Group V, HIV+ and AIDS patients

Type of Group	Objectives	Initiative	Training	Method
Prostitutes	Accept status	Love	Doctors	1 to 1 counselling
Blood recipients	-also within family	Safe sex	Nurses	Group counselling
IV drug users	Positive outlook	Dangers of repeat infections	AIDS counsellors	Positive media
Jail inmates	Receive regular counselling	Counsel concerns	Self help groups	-films
Spouses	Receive medical treatment	Maintain positive outlook	Parent/family groups	Help lines
Others	Financial support	Meet financial/ social concerns	Peer groups	Meditation
	Information on medical treatment	Hygiene	Religious groups/ leaders	
	-allopathic homoeo, ayurveda		AIDS rights activists	
	Information on rights		Village leaders/elders	
	Sexual education			
	Job placement			
	Dietary planning			
	Risk situations			
	- avoid opp. infections			
	- hygiene			
	Counsel families			
	Educate on disease progression			
	Spiritual guidance			
	Family concerns-financial,			
	-social			
	Support groups			
	Help phones			
	Meditation/ relaxation			
	Crisis management			
	Love			

Information, Education

6.6 Positive Media

Positive media is a necessary step towards educating the public towards understanding the disease and how to protect themselves. It has been very unfortunate that the vast majority of media and public health education have used scare tactics in an effort to raise attention towards the modes of infection. However, as has been observed in more developed countries, these tactics fail and often go on to create the stigma that is present. Further to this, public health efforts such as the awareness campaign by the health department for the township of Anand cause endless detriment towards the understanding of this disease by creating and perpetuating the AIDS DEMON. The media should be directed towards specific groups in a manner that will be accepted. One such example of decent efforts in the direction was in Bombay on November 29th/99 when music was used to draw attention of truck drivers. A concert was organized by NGO Population Services International (PSI). Using song and dance, the organization hoped to get the attention of the truck drivers. This system obviously created results, as after the show the queue for condoms and proper information extended several hundred metres[lxxx].

Another example of positive media awareness can be displayed in Tamil Nadu, where local TV advertisements appeal to men through a common denominator, cricket. The advertising reads "*If you go out tonight and bowl over a maiden, use a condom*".

Chapter 7

EMPOWERMENT

7.1 Positive (+) People

One long term survivor of HIV has said *"for those of us residing in the kingdom of the sick it is hard to explain to those who are healthy that hope is like the air that we breathe, it is essential to survival"* [lxxxi].

Psychoneuroimmunology has come up with the notion that *"positive coping"* is a crucial factor in survival. But positive coping is not only the focusing on the positive, it is also avoiding the negative. Solomon and Temoshok (the originators of PNI) suggest that survival includes:

1) An acceptance of the diagnosis without the belief that HIV is an automatic death sentence.

2) Willingness to take responsibility for their own healing and make major life changes.

3) A passionate commitment to life, a sense of the meaning and purpose of life, an ability to identify goals.

4) A good, open, healing relationship between themselves and their healthcare providers, being neither passively compliant, nor reactively defiant.

5) Meeting and talking with other people with AIDS in a supportive environment, getting and giving information and support, being altruistically involved with other people with HIV.
6) Being assertive.
7) A sensitivity towards their own needs and a willingness to nurture themselves.
8) Physical exercise.
9) An ability to communicate openly about concerns.
10) A personalized means of coping that is believed to have beneficial health effects.[lxxxii]

For some time, in several developed countries, HIV/AIDS acted as a somewhat fashionable disease. The carriers were seen as 'martyrs' of certain communities. This is certainly not the case in developing nations, however, it may be said that the patient and loved ones may learn and experience happiness not previously present in their lives. This may sound strange, however, many patients begin to appreciate the world around them as they prepare for death, or rather, life with a sure end. A love of life and sincere desire to live life to its fullest can be observed, even in the most unlikely patients. Let us consider the case of 'Raju', who had received notice of his infection in front of a crowd that ridiculed him. Raju had previously been a drug addict, an alcoholic, and visited prostitutes; however, Raju had also received a blood transfusion after an accident. After diagnosis, Raju turned his back on his old ways and says that he now lives life to the fullest as a counsellor helping other HIV+ individuals. Raju explains that he has found happiness a and reason to live which he had previously not felt[lxxxiii].

The disease often gives people permission to do things that they previously would not have considered. It can make it easier to say 'no' to unwelcome stresses, duties, jobs, or demands. It can serve as permission to do what one has always wanted to do but has been 'too busy' to start. It can allow the individual the time to reflect, meditate, and decide on their future. The disease can serve as an excuse for misgivings. It can make it easier to express and accept love, to speak of ones feelings. The smallest flower may now appear beautiful when previously the entire tree may have been a drab.

It is necessary that the patient be taught to focus on these positives and not to dwell on the negative effects of the potential disease. If the individual can be empowered to develop positive attitudes towards their state there is a much better opportunity for the health care provider to help, and in turn, have the individual help others, whether it be the immediate family or other PLWHA.

7.2 Familial Empowerment

It is an Indiah tradition that families live together in the same house, one generation with another generation. Therefore it is not surprising that the majority of PLWHA do so in a familial surrounding. There are however, detriments to this. As has been observed, occasionally the family will not accept the patient and will banish them from the house. The shocking case of a patient being kept outside by his family exemplifies this, as they believed that his disease was a punishment for his lifestyle. Other cases of the family not accepting the patient is when the patient is a CSW; the family will often banish them or ridicule them into leaving. The blame attached to the disease is apparent, as more than half of the cases examined are as a result of infidelity. It is an unfortunate reality that often the spouse is an equal victim of the promiscuity, and thus causes anger and resentment, understandably.

However, the family can also be a wonderful asset for the patient, particularly in later life, as they often act as the health care givers and counsellors. The family must be taught to become accepting of the PLWHA, they must be taught to deliver non-judgmental support. The field team must be able to teach the families the proper care methods of the individual, along with care for themselves.. The families are informed that the virus is spread through bodily fluids and so it is necessary to explain the proper methods of waste disposal and hygiene of the individual.

The family must become the counsellor for the patient and remove blame. Obviously this is difficult when a spouse is infected as a result of extra- marital affairs, however, both individuals are patients and so must receive respect. Unfortunately, in the cases where a child is infected it is difficult to console the mother, but attempts must be made.

Most extended families are accepting of their relatives health status and do much to help. They are often the only source of economic stability towards later life, and provide food, clothing, and shelter, to the PLWHA. It is necessary to provide counselling to the families periodically, and particularly after the patient, or the patients die.

Familial care goes beyond providing an effective and practical solution to the paucity of existing resources; it becomes a potent weapon for improving the quality of life of the PLWHA, the family, and the community[lxxxiv].

Community Empowerment:

Support from the community implies that the community is aware of the virus, takes steps to insure that it does not spread, supports families caring for PLWHA and provides care directly to the PLWHA. It facilitates a positive atmosphere for the patient, family and community where mutual reciprocal interactions abound. Myths and misconceptions, discrimination and barriers, are broken down.

The concept of the social stigma attached to HIV and AIDS is as pandemic as the disease itself. However, we too, would be stereotyping if we expected to find prejudice so rampant. It was therefore, a pleasant surprise at times to visit rural villages in Gujarat and talk to the local people of their attitudes or knowledge about HIV (See photos 1.6 &1.8). Many of the villagers knew little about the disease but admitted that they thought that it was prevalent in their villages and certainly the spread should be stopped. The majority of villagers have received no formal education, but does not mean that they are ignorant. The general attitude in the villages was welcoming the education, as the elders worried for the future of the young. Often the villagers were aware that the disease is spread through sexual contact, however know little else. Knowledge of safe sex practices is uncommon, but welcomed. The elders of the villages can be most relied upon to make decisions for the community, and so, it has been necessary to gain their acceptance. This was not best accomplished as appearing as a group of outsiders, with the obvious foreigners; rather this was best achieved through being introduced by villagers who may already be known to the hospital staff. The villagers known to the staff acted as initial intermediaries between the field team and elders. This manner enabled trust and acceptance, making meetings with the elders easier. The elders of the villages were concerned about the future health of the young, as they were aware that it is now common place for younger males to use prostitutes. Therefore, the elders encouraged organizing public rallies to gain awareness for their people. It was certainly encouraging to be invited so quickly to teach the groups, as one may have expected a defense. However, public rallies can often be a waste of time; as the villagers come out simply to see the outsiders and the foreigners, and then go back to the normal routine.

It was therefore necessary to organize teams of educators for focus group discussions as a part of the day long rallies. Each team of 2-3 field team members would visit the houses of families and discuss HIV and STD's with them. This method would eventually reach all people in the village as those in smaller homes would come and watch the lessons at the houses of bigger families. The responses were generally good, and often any denial of a problem in the community was countered by an argument from another community member, thus creating dialogue and more information.

The topics discussed included safe sex with unmarried persons, and with prostitutes. Blood transfusion was also discussed as this is a common method of infection, and so, the villagers were encouraged to use government hospitals, with tested blood. Also discussed was the treatment of HIV+ individuals, explaining that they were no different from the other villagers and so should be treated equally in the village. The team attempted to convey the message that their role was as a health partner with the village; to help the village deal with challenges. The elders of the village were asked to find volunteers who would be willing to help with chores for the PLWHA; so as to encourage community involvement and intersectoral collaboration. This involved having those with available resources to help out where it was needed most. Examples of this were the men and women who had worked in a health care setting, such as hospital porters; also those with vehicles; and those with ample food supplies.

Having approached the group in such a manner, it has been possible to grasp what are the *Strengths, Weaknesses, Opportunities, and Threats* of the villagers. With so many villages in the area surrounding. Anand it is not possible for the field team to care and teach everyone, so the community must take responsibility for its health.

Survey:

To properly display the lack of understanding and attitudes of the general population in western India it has been necessary to conduct a survey. The survey consisted of two large groups: 100 HIV+ individuals and 200 individuals of the general population with no consideration towards their health status. The questionnaires were in English, Hindi, and Gujarati.

7.5 Survey 1

Table 12. Survey 1 : General Population

Age groups	Percentage of those surveyed
0- 20	12%
21-30	42%
31-40	23%
41-50	16%
51 and above	7%

The questions were in a simple yes/no style so as to be able to ascertain statistics. One question, question two, required answers, however, for the purpose of the statistics it will be assumed that the answer was either answered completely or not. The survey was conducted in October 1999 in Anand, Gujarat. The gender of all participants is male as the females refused to take part. The majority of those questioned were between the ages of 21-30, which is the higher risk group for transmission of HIV infection.

Q 1 : Do you think that HIV/AIDS is a problem in your community?

Statistical Answer : 52% No

48% Yes

Q 2 : Do you know anyone suffering from HIV/ AIDS in your community?

Statistical Answer : 100% No

Q 3 : Describe two ways in which a person may become infected with HIV/AIDS?

Statistical Answer: 73% answered the question correctly and completely

27% answered incompletely or not at all

Q 4 : Do you think that HIV/AIDS is a punishment?

Statistical Answer: 62% Yes

38% No or left unanswered

Q 5 : Do you believe that there is a cure for HIV/AIDS?

Statistical Answer: 19% Yes

81% No or left unanswered

The results of this survey clearly indicate that the regional public health authorities are providing poor information about HIV/AIDS. The answers to question 1 indicate that the general population is unaware of the disease in the community, even though the major towns Anand and Baroda, have large numbers of HIV carriers and post-HIV deaths; similarly, almost every small village has individuals carrying the disease. It is not surprising that the answer to question 2 was 100% negative, as it is unlikely that those knowing a positive person or being positive themselves would reveal this to a stranger. It is, however, most alarming that the answers to question 3 revealed that almost one third of those asked were unable to describe two modes of infection; it is likely that a greater proportion would be unable to describe a third route of transmission. Question number 4 was necessary to ask as it would reveal the superstition and misguidance that is so regularly held. A startling 62% of those surveyed answered that they believed the disease was a punishment to the individual. Further questioning would be necessary to determine if this belief is linked to religion or not. To gather the general perception of medical treatment through public health education, superstition, and tales; question number 5 displayed that almost 1/5th of those asked believed that there was a cure for HIV/AIDS. Again, further questioning would be necessary to discover if this cure were through medical, whether allopathic, ayurvedic, homoeopathic,etc., or through spiritual facilities. In conclusion, this survey sufficiently indicates that a greater drive towards awareness and education is necessary on the part of the local public health board.

7.6 Survey 2: HIV+ve individuals

The second survey to be conducted involved a group of 100 HIV+ individuals, in the states of Gujarat and Maharashtra. The questions were asked in a simple manner so as to enable all of the participants to clearly answer. It is unlikely that all of the questions were answered in truth by all individuals, particularly those relating to the patients sexual history.

However, it is questions 2, 3, 4, and 5 which are pertinent to this study. The questionnaires were in English, Gujarati, Hindi, and Marathi. The gender of the groups were almost equal (57% male, 43% female).

Table 13. HIV+ Individuals

Age groups	Percentage of those surveyed
15-20	17%
21-30	41%
31-40	38%
51-50	4%
51 and above	0%

Q 1 : Do you feel that HIV/AIDS is a punishment for past experiences?

Statistical answer: 44% Yes

56% No

Q 2 : Do you feel that you are receiving adequate medical treatment?

Statistical answer: 21% Yes

79% No

Q 3 : Have you considered ayurveda or homoeopathic treatment?

Statistical answer: 36% Yes

64% No

Empowerment 65

Q 4 : Would you be willing to receive ayurveda or homoeopathy if your doctor recommended?
Statistical answer: 82%Yes
18%No

Q 5 : How long do you expect to remain healthy?
Statistical answer: Up to 10 years- 69%
More than 10 years- 22%
No answer- 9%

The results of the second survey indicate that the HIV+ individuals have many opinions on their health. The answers indicate that the patients have not got much control over their health decisions and are looking for the guidance of their health provider. In question 1, 44% of the group responded that they did indeed feel that the HIV infection was a punishment for their past actions. It would take a separate study to determine if these anxieties were based upon religious or moral issues. It is, however, necessary to note that it is likely more than 44% feel this way. Counselling and support are obviously necessary to dispel this myth within the individuals. The answer to question 2 reveals that these individuals are well aware that they are not receiving the best treatment possible. Many individuals inquire about antir-etroviral drugs and are immediately told that as they cannot afford them there is no way to receive them. It should also be mentioned that very few specialists in HIV infection are present in India. Question 3 reveals that a small amount (36%) of those questioned have attempted to find other treatment in ayurveda and homoeopathy. Further to this, question 4 displays the obvious control that the healthcare provider has as an advisor: 82% have said that they would consider ayurveda or homoeopathy if recommended, this would obviously be beneficial as both therapies concentrate on neuroimmunilogical status. The final question, which may seem crude, was necessary as it divides the group into those who accept the prognosis and life expectancy given to them by their health provider or education group, to those that wish to defy the odds and expect to lead a normal life, despite being labelled as diseased.

■■

Chapter 8

TREATMENT

8.1 Conventional/Allopathic Medicine

At present there is no cure for HIV infection or AIDS. A number of drugs have been created which can suppress the HIV progression, thus improving longevity of life. More recently, protease inhibitors, have managed to check the progression of the disease resulting in extended lifespan prognosis and increasing the quality of life. The drugs neither restore the immune system nor destroy the HIV already in the cells. Many individuals suffer side effects as a result of the intense chemotherapy; anemia, nausea, malaise, insomnia, depression, and even as serious as hepatitis and prominent skeletal features result from the drug regimen. Many patients take as many as 26 tablets per day, often to counteract the side effects of others. While this is by no means condemning the scientific and ethical breakthroughs that have come about through these drugs, we must wonder if they can, at times, cause as much damage as good.

Nevertheless, the expensive drug regimes can be called an opulent luxury of living in developed countries, such as Canada, U.K., Scandinavia, where the government is willing to provide the drugs to the patients. It may well be suggested that the larger pharmaceutical corporations are overlooking their charitable duties by demanding the high prices for the desired drugs. Rarely can these drug regimens be afforded in developing countries. In India, the drug AZT costs a monthly 30'000Rs ($1050 CAN), impossible for an the average HIV patient who earns a monthly 1000Rs ($35 CAN). For the few who do manage to acquire the money, the length of time that they receive the drugs can put themselves and their families into financial ruin. It is for this reason that a cost- effective alternative must be found.

The standard care in developed nations for PLWHA is combination therapy using multiple antiretroviral drugs. This is normally initiated with one protease inhibitor and two reverse transcriptase inhibitors, once the CD4+ T lymphocyte count is less than 500 /uL, or the patient is symptomatic. It is assumed that the best results are found if the combination therapy is started early and aggressively. Therapy can bring CD4 counts up substantially from very low levels. However, as has been noticed, new syndromes associated with the immune restabilization are appearing, thus long term results may be detrimental. Many of the newer drugs have unknown side effects that can themselves be devastating. For example, Indinavir can result in renal calculi, hyperbillirubinemia, and abdominal pains; Ritinovir, statistically showing the highest incidence of side effects, has been linked to nausea, vomiting, diarrhoea, fatigue, circumoral paresthesias, anorexia, elevated triglyceride, creatinine, and transaminases levels; little is known about Nelfinavir[lxxxvi].

For the wealthy few who can afford antiretroviral drugs in the likes of India, combinations are not a possibility. The luxury of financial access to anti-retroviral drugs is limited to the above mentioned drugs, normally used in monotherapy. It is observed that in monotherapy, drug resistance is inevitable. Major trials by the Concorde group[lxxxvii, lxxxviii] and the AIDS Clinical Trials Group (ACTG) 019 protocol[lxxxix] have shown that the benefit of monotherapy in delaying disease progression in asymptomatic patients was small and temporary.

8.2 Ayurvedic Medicine

Ayurvedic medicine is not often understood in the western world and it is often the case that it receives undue respect as people simply assume that as it has stood the test of time, surely it is a substantial therapy.

Ayurveda has been practiced in India for several thousand years and is believed to be a system of medicine derived from the gods. Ayurvedic doctors attend school for five and a half years, learning subjects such as anatomy, physiology, pathology, pharmacology, and surgery, as well as their various therapies. Ayurveda is based on the therapy of cleansing the body and then allowing for balancing to occur.

Ayurveda translates literally to "the knowledge of long life". Practitioners of this wisdom are called *Vaidyas*. Ayurveda takes a holistic approach to diagnosis where mental and emotional symptoms are as important as physical. Ayurveda is associated with maintaining a balance between the three bodily essences or doshas, *vatta (wind-air and space), pitta (bile- fire and water), and kapha (phlegm- earth and water)*. Vatta represents kinetic energy and is associated with the nervous system and movement. Kapha, which opposes vatta, is potential energy and is associated with lymph and mucous. Pitta mediates between these two forces, governing digestive and metabolic processes. Balance between the three doshas is essential to

Table 14 : Antiretroviral Therapy

Drug	Indication	Dose	Common Side Effects	Monitoring
Zididuvine (AZT)	CD4 < 300/uL or symptomatic disease	500-600mg orally in divided doses	Anemia, neutropaenia, nausea malaise, headache, insomnia	CBC every 3 months
Didanosine (DDI)	Intolerance to AZT or combined with AZT	125-300mg orally tbd.	Peripheral neuropathy, pancreatitis hepatitis	CBC and differential aminotransferases, potassium, amylase, triglycerides, & monthly neurologic exams.
Zalcitabine (ddC)	Intolerance to AZT or combined with AZT	0.375-0.75mg orally bd.	Peripheral neuropathy, aphtous ulcerations, hepatitis	Monthly neurologic exams
Staduvine (d4T)	CD4 <300/uL and intolerant to AZT/ DDI/ ddC	40-60mg oral/v daily	Peripheral neuropathy, hepatitis pancreatitis	Monthly neurologic exams, amylase test, aminotransferases

Source:PDR[lxxxv]

good health, but decadent doshas unbalanced by *Agni (fire)* develop distortions.

Ayurvedic doctors claim that the disease AIDS has been mentioned in the "Sharangdhar Samhita", an ancient sanskrit manuscript by his Highness Sharangdhar. The name of the disease in the book is "Oja Kisha", and is related to AIDS by virtue of its symptoms, here the reference relates to a disease of kings. The method of treatment for this ailment varies, however, inevitably involves *Panchekarma*. *Panchekarma* is a system of therapies developed to cleanse the body of all impurities, therefore balancing doshas. The different modalities used include induced vomiting, enemas, intense steam, massage, leeching, and shaving the head to allow absorption of medicated oils (See photos 3.1,3.2,.3.3, & 3.4). Many side effects are noted in Panchekarma. The patient will later receive oral medicaments and dietary restrictions. Of the cases that I observed in the J.S. Ayurvedic Hospital in Nadiad, Gujarat, few were receiving considerable benefit. It was also interesting to note that a medical system that purports to have a history of dealing with AIDS, this hospital refused admission to HIV+ patients for the In-Patients Department (IPD).

Various combinations of herbs, minerals, and elements are used in the Ayurvedic preparations for boosting the health of PLWHA. 38 different remedies were used in an immunity boosting preparation by a group of Ayurvedic physicians in Karnataka. This preparation costs the patients Rs 1575 ($56 CAN) per month, plus an additional Rs 500 ($17 CAN) per litre of oil used in deep massage panchakarma. Ayurveda is a costly treatment but appears to have some efficacy in relieving symptoms in the patients. Research has been sponsored by the WHO in Ayurveda at a hospital in Junagaht, Gujarat; however, no results have yet been published.

There are reports of Ayurvedic doctors in Kerala, south India, who specialize in HIV treatment, and, for a fee, will heal the patient. Another example of creating false hope in the patients can best be demonstrated in the example provided (See following page) related to advertising "vaccine therapy" using an ancient medical system; further to this the alleged doctor can organize marriage, and apparently much more, after completely curing the patient. Obviously, these reports are based more on the fraudulent acts than on health; however, as the patients are often grasping for any treatment they may rely upon the quacks. Another such case was observed in the clinic of Dr. P.C. Dave of Vadodara, as a patient presenting with a "moon- face" told that she was taking ayurvedic medicines; however, when Dr. Dave had the tablets tested at a laboratory, the medicaments contained ayurvedic medicines combined with steroids. The harshness of even the ayurvedic tablets, which are often derived from metals, making them difficult on the liver, kidneys, and pancreas, can have severe side effects. It is unlikely that ayurveda can provide much relief in the treatment of HIV and panchakarma will likely cause more harm than good; as the patients immune systems are compromised, they can hardly tolerate the purging effects of 15- 16 cycles of vomiting.

8.3 Homoeopathy

Homoeopathy was founded 200 years ago by a German physician Dr. Christian Samuel Hahnemann. Homoeopathy is based on Hanemann's concept "similia similibus curentur" (let like cure like)[xc]. Homoeopathy began with the experiments of Hahnemann on the effects of cinchona bark (quinine) once ingested. In a series of repeated tests, Hahnemann observed certain pathological effects, which appeared to resemble intermittent fever. Enthused with the experiments, Hahnemann studied many other substances. This led Hahnemann to establish a new concept of cure by the use of substances, which are capable of creating such disturbances in healthy human beings, by the use of the same substance in smaller doses. This marked the formal beginning of homoeopathy in 1796. Homoeopathy considers the entire individual's mental, emotional, and physical symptoms and treats the sum of symptoms according to the concept of simile. It is the aim of homoeopathy to produce a reactivation, or stimulation of the auto- regulatory activity in the organism, strengthening the system. In this sense it plays a preventive and promotive role for health.

In 1993, the *British Homoeopathic* Journal published a study conducted by the Central Council for Homoeopathy in India from 1989 to 1991. The study involving the homoeopathic treatment of 129 asymptomatic patients was qualitative concluding that 12 patients converted to HIV-ve within one year of treatment[xci]. A further double-blind placebo study was conducted by the CCRH in 1999; the study revealed a relatively significant difference between pre-and post-haematological levels in the verum group, whilst those of the placebo group yielded non- significant results (See table 15)[xcii]. It is for this reason that I travelled to Mumbai in August of 1999 to interview Dr. Vikram Singh. Dr Singh informed me that while no other patients have reverted back to HIV-ve, many continue to do well and maintain health. We can conclude from this that as no patients have reverted back to HIV-ve in the past eight years that these patients were likely originally tested with false positives. However, as Western Blot testing was never done to conclude the situations we must assume that the spot tests are unreliable. Further to this, the double- blind placebo trial rendered only relatively significant results. The CCRH rely strictly upon homoeopathic treatment and no counselling or exercise regimes are recommended. It is likely that homoeopathy can benefit the patient more significantly when combined with a healthy regimen of counselling, diet, exercise, and meditation.

It is impossible to suggest that we will be able to remove the organism from the body. Dr. Singh suggests that he is prolonging life, maintaining health , totally free of cost. The allopathic drugs in India are so very expensive and have many side effects, such as anemia, emesis, skin problems, which in turn require more drugs, and therefore more money. Homoeopathy may be able to provide an alternative to those that have none.

The studies conducted by the CCRH, as well as the attached original study (See Annexure I), suggest that homoeopathy may play a role in the treatment of HIV+ve patients, particularly as a cost effective option.

Drug Prophylaxis:

CCR5 or CC-CKr-5, is a cell chemikine receptor on the surface of the T-lymphocyte acting as a co-receptor for HIV in the initial infection period. Another membrane bound receptor, CXCR4 (or fusin) can be dominant in later stages of HIV infection. Both of the receptors act to guide the HIV to access the CD4+ lymphocyte[xciv, xcv]. It has been known for some years that some individuals are not developing infection despite repeated exposure, and that some patients develop the disease extremely slowly. The statistics reveal that as many as 1% of the white population is homozygous for the defect in the CCR5 receptor (due to delta-32 gene), and as many as 15% are heterozygous for a defect. It is assumed then, that those homozygous individuals are immune to the viral replication, and

Table 15 : Descriptive Characteristics at the end of CCRH Double Blind Study

Placebo	Verum (n=18)	Parameter (n=20)	P value
Body weight	53.61	53.30	0.74
previously	53.39	52.95	
CD4 T- lymphocytes	452.00	534.35	0.52
previously	443.61	433.30	
CD8 T- lymphocytes	1298.50	1327.25	0.98
previously	1256.89	1234.20	
Haemoglobin	12.73	12.40	0.96
previously	12.77	12.89	
Haematocrit	39.38	38.59	0.83
previously	39.58	40.20	
White Blood Corpuscles (WBC)	6744.44	6410.00	0.66
previously	7222.22	6550.00	
Source: CCRH[xciii]			

that the heterozygous population, may only develop the infection slowly. This information has thus opened a new field for study in genetics. If it would be possible to detect the CCR5 in the general population, it may be possible to prevent infection. If those already infected were to receive receptor altering drugs, then the disease progression may be slowed[xcvi]. Thus till now, allopathic prophylaxis is not available on a wide spectrum. It is, however, likely available in cases of presumed exposure, of course, to the lucky few. The approach to prophylaxis immediately after exposure can reduce transmission by up to 90%, using AZT. In wealthy healthcare areas, two anti-retroviral drugs along with one protease inhibitor are normally administered for 1 month. Although the likelihood of infection through needlestick is low, the treatment is recommended. However, side effects exist.

Homoeopathy has proven to be of great benefit in preventing a particular disease in treated individuals during epidemics. An interesting situation arose in December 1999 in the region of Hospet, Karnataka, India, when, during an epidemic of Japanese encephalitis, the homoeopathic remedy Belladonna 200c was given to 11'000 children. Note the case of Guaratingueta in Brazil 1974, when during a meningitis outbreak 18,640 children were administered the homoeopathic remedy Meningococcinum 10c, whilst a remaining 6,340 did not receive the nosode. Of the children in the homoeopathic group only four cases of meningitis occurred, of the latter untreated group thirty four cases were noted[xcvii].

Certainly it can be said that HIV is presently pandemic. The consideration however, as to whether prophylaxis against the Human Immunodeficiency Virus has yet to be justly considered. In the past, homoeopathic preparations regarding epidemics have been successful, but they have invariably been used in acute and intense diseases, i.e. scarlet fever, cholera, pertussis; all of which epidemics have affected many people with similar development of symptoms. This allowed for selection of remedies characteristic to the given disease, or a choice of a *genus epidemicus*. The genus epidemicus is a near specific remedy chosen having examined many cases and observed similarities between the majority. However this method is only useful when there is a clear threat to the health of the population. This method could not be applied for the prophylaxis of HIV as HIV is not an acute disease, and the manifestations tend to be very different in different patients. It is only in the latter stages that the similarities between symptoms are occasionally observed.

The method of prophylaxis by prescription of constitutional remedies has proven efficacious in the past regarding epidemics and childhood infections. This method however, has not been examined in the case of HIV as it would be necessary to have patients under treatment who we know contracted the infection whilst under good homoeopathic treatment. This is unlikely as we cannot be sure that the treatment was correct, or that the patient became infected whilst under treatment.

Homoeopathic prophylaxis using a disease product such as the nosode *Pertussinum* in the avoidance of pertussis has proven to be efficacious. However, treatment using a potentized HIV would likely be unhelpful as it is often not the virus that is the sickness, rather it is the opportunistic infections that cause sickness. There is not presently a proving of the HIV or AIDS nosode that can be trusted as the proving performed is an embarrassment to homoeopathy; and an offense to PLWHA. The provers involved did not ingest the remedy, made from the blood of an expired AIDS patient. Further to this, the drug proved was not truly a nosode as nosodes are made of morbid matter, as is the case with Psorinum (a scabies vescicle), Medhorrhinum (a gonorrheal discharge), Lueticum (a spirochete in a syphilitic discharge), Tuberculinum (a Koch exotoxin), Carcinosinum (cancerous breast tissue), etc..

HIV is a chronic infection, but not necessarily a chronic disease as we are aware that there are many people living healthy lives after years of infection. Therefore, developing a homoeopathic prophylaxis against the virus is unlikely, however, the aforementioned constitutional treatment and combination therapy may lessen susceptibility to opportunistic infections as the immune system will hopefully remain healthy.

Chapter 9

HOMOEOPATHY

9.1 Indications for homoeopathic observations

PLWHA live in a perpetual state of fear, not so much of dying, but of being rejected by society if their HIV status becomes known to others. Rejection is often linked to a feeling of extreme anxiety and helplessness, a fear that their life is finished. Understanding how important the attitude of the physician is in the overall health of the patient, the patient will often be observing the attitude of the physician to grade hope. This observation can be as disheartening or disillusioning as a low CD4+ count. Over time, and with decent counselling, this may change. The counsellor, whether health care provider or not, can help the individual to view HIV infection as something to live with, rather than die from. The best example of this in practice is the Salvation Army, Mumbai HIV/AIDS unit, who have a counsellor named "Tony" (not his real name). Tony has been HIV+ since 1992; he has felt the shame and social abuse and can now counsel the other individuals to overcome this, and enjoy life to its fullest, "even more than HIV negative people" claims Tony[xcviii].

When dealing with the patient, it is necessary to listen closely to them and also observe the changes in their bodies. One of the best things that a health care worker can do is be there, to listen, and by listening, encourage the person to talk about their feelings, let them know that you care. Often the patients have heard unprofessional advice and recommendations, so the professional should talk this out with the patient to deal with questions. Remember that the patient has already received a lot of advice and criticism, so simply listening is the most important job of a care worker, whether health professional or not. However sick someone is, they can still be included in daily duties giving them a place in their environment. The need for love and acceptance from the care worker is particularly important, especially for people who are experiencing loneliness, isolation, and rejection. People having HIV are at a crucial point in their lives, where death is ominous and even the health care worker is *momento more*. People approaching the end of life may find that decent counselling can help them to accept and understand what is happening. It is possible that they will deny their illness, or become angry and blameful. They may despair at the absence of cure, be anxious about partners or family, feel grief and guilt. It is useful for the individual to be put into contact with others in a similar situation, so recommending to put the individual in contact with a local support group is advisable.

People with HIV may need spiritual support. They may feel cut off from their religion or religious community. Some people find it beneficial to talk with others of a similar faith, or to practice their religion even if they have not done so in a long time. This may be of concern for the homoeopathic prescription and so listening intently is necessary. However, others may feel pressured into talking about religious issues when they would prefer not to. Care workers should acknowledge a person's spiritual beliefs or lack thereof, and respect this choice.

9.2 Selecting the remedy

Selecting the remedy in cases of HIV should be on a constitutional basis, that is, to consider the mental, emotional, physical, and pathological symptoms, including life history. This is an ideal situation which is however, not always available. It is often the case that the patient will present with an advanced stage of the disease or after much use of suppressive and toxic drugs. The use of suppressive drugs unfortunately makes the task of finding a single matching remedy difficult as the characteristic and peculiar symptoms are often no longer present. In such cases it may be only possible to palliate.

Patients that present at an aysmptomatic stage, before chemotherapies, have the best prognosis for maintaining health. Constitutional treatment considering mental, emotional, and physical symptoms should be regularly monitored and, in a perfect situation, have regular blood investigations. Intercurrent remedies, such as nosodes, may be employed occasionally over time. During this period the susceptibility of the patient should be quite high and it is the job of the homoeopath to maintain it so.

Patients that present in a progressive state of the disease should be carefully attended to. Often the immune system is unstable and can be highly reactive to all drugs, even homoeopathy. As a result, it is often best to begin such cases with low to moderate potencies, repeatedly. It is most often that the patient had received allopathic symptomatic treatment for their complaints and thus the true symptomatology is not present. The immune system is weakened and not displaying its characteristic and peculiar symptoms. Hence it may be necessary to begin with indicated remedies. (See Annexure II).

The general symptoms of the patient will best indicate the progress of health or disease. Pay particular attention to the energy level of the patient, note fatigue if present. Appetite is a good indication of health and also remedy, note the desires and aversions, and any change in appetite. Pay close attention to the passage of urine, frequency, and color or clarity. A very indicative feature of the disease progression are the glandular swellings of the lymph in the cervical and axilliary regions; we shall call this the "four lymph region" (2 pairs). Note which sides are most affected for prescribing. At the stage of generalized persistent lymphadenopathy we must be aware of what we are hoping for homoeopathy to do, as often when the swelling goes down and we see this as a good sign, it is in fact, that the infection is no longer being fought and the patient will likely experience a deterioration in health. Examine skin eruptions for those that are HIV related, note shingles, herpes zoster, dermatitis, epiditis, or ringworm infections. The skin eruptions may be a good indicator of health and remedy choice. Note that itching cannot always be relied upon as a symptom of HIV as it may be related secondarily due to persistent sweating or weather changes, sodium attaching to the hair follicles causing irritation. Attention must be paid to sleep and sleep patterns. Sleep is often reduced as the progression of the disease continues. Pay attention to the dreams of the patients, these may indicate how the patient is coping with the disease and may lead to miasm or remedy choice. For example, if the patient is complaining of frightening dreams, it may be due to the fact that he is dwelling on the disease; note that sycotic and tubercular patients cover up their fears, but the frightening dreams indicate that the fears are inescapable. Body weight is perhaps the best indicator of how the individuals disease is progressing. There are three parameters used for assessing the weight loss: 1- more than 10% of original body weight;

2- up to 30%; and 3- up to 50%. Pay close attention to fevers as these are a good indication of a remedy. Tuberculosis, pneumonitis, pneumocystis carinii, pulmonary coughs are very common complications in HIV. Even if the person has developed pneumonia it must be directly linked to the tubercular diathesis. Pulmonary complaints must be dealt with very swiftly, if homoeopathically, particularly in larger cities, due to pollution. It is at this time that allopathy is often called upon to intervene or we can expect a quick deterioration and unexpected death. During the last few days or hours of a persons life the health care worker should focus on minimizing distress and maintaining respect. It can be difficult to tell when death is near, but it is important not to leave the patient alone, as many people are afraid of dying alone. It is wise to remember that hearing is normally the last sense left before death, so encourage family and loved ones to talk compassionately to the individual.

9.3 Prescribing

The choice of remedies is obviously the most important job of the homoeopath. The remedy decision should be based on clearly comprehensible method, not on key note, nor whimsical prescribing. If the homoeopath is prone to theorizing on a case, perhaps the HIV cases should be passed to a more experienced homoeopath. Each case must be viewed individually, not related to other cases of similar pathology. The homoeopath must have taken an adequate case and used clearly perceivable methods in the decision, using repertorial and materia medica knowledge. Remember that the patient is reaching out to the homoeopath for help, and so, a lack of knowledge or bias is not an excuse to give an incorrectly chosen remedy. A solid knowledge of the materia medica is necessary, not only that of the polychrests or the commonly used drugs. Using methods such as a pendulum or radionics to achieve the remedy is not homoeopathy and this should be explained to the patient. It is necessary to clearly understand the pathology of the case and allow the prescription to follow the pathology. If we believe that the mental symptoms are the most important symptoms in a case then we must also agree that the physical symptoms follow or correspond to the mental/ emotional symptoms; thus maintaining that the physical symptoms cannot be overlooked.

If the case has not progressed to a symptomatic phase then the prognosis may be good. Homoeopathy may be said to work best in maintaining health and maintaining immunity. At this time the constitutional drug, or remedy most fitting the general physical symptoms and mental and emotional symptoms has to be given. It may be necessary to differentiate miasms at this time to help in remedy selection. The constitutional drug is most often found through careful roportorizing of the caco and then thorough oxamination of the materia medica. A good homoeopath will be able to prescribe well at this time. However, we cannot assume that the constitutional drug will always act wonders; while it may be a similimum, it may not affect the patient rapidly enough. Often the constitutional remedy will act over a long period of time, improving health, which is obviously what is required in cases of HIV. The body's healing mechanism is compromised to varying degrees and so must be stimulated gently. Empirical evidence has shown that the remedies will best act in an HIV carrying individual in medium to lower potencies. Higher potencies, particularly initially, may be a shock to the system. Many remedies are too deep acting to use in high potencies to begin with; also, if the homoeopath is unsure of pathological state, a high potency may be detrimental, as is the case with Lycopodium or Phosphorus.

The debatable subject of single remedy, single dose, must be called into play often in the cases of HIV. It is likely that the constitutional drug will heighten the health of the individual, but what to do when the opportunistic infections or ailments appear; if the constitutional drug is already acting, then it may do little. Remedies affecting specific ailments or *specifics* may be necessary here. The term specific is a misnomer here as it will still need to be verified in the materia medica to be homoeopathic to the case.

Nosodes are of immense importance in the cases of HIV and often appear to be the most indicated remedies. This is arguably due to the fact that the disease is weakening the body's natural disease fighting capabilities and allowing innate disease to appear. The prescription of nosodes in the cases cannot be routine, rather should be based on sound principles and only used if homoeopathic or the most indicated remedy fails to act. However, evidence has shown that the prescription of nosodes as intercurrent remedies has proven to be the most efficient approach. It has been suggested that the case may be started with a miasmatic approach, by giving nosodes, to the point of a drug aggravation being induced, to arouse the system. However, this opinion has also been harshly criticized as mixing the case. With regard to the notion that the indicated remedy fails to act, the homoeopath must initially have humility and wonder if the remedy was, in fact, the similimum. It is most likely that the miasmatic approach, using nosodes as an intercurrent remedy would be most indicated during the early symptomatic phase. Careful study of the dominant miasm will allow for the selection of a nosode.

Knowledge of all remedies is necessary while prescribing for HIV cases. Therefore the use of sound repertories is necessary, such as Kent's, Phatak's, Synthesis, Complete, etc. The homoeopath must learn when to prescribe the indicated remedy. Often the constitutional drug may be apparent, but will not react as quickly as a homoeopathic fast acting remedy. Similarly, the patient may require an extremely low potency of a remedy, possibly as an organ support or as a fortifier. Remedies such a Alfalfa or Hydrastis Canadensis are indispensable in progressive HIV infection. Other remedies such as Avena Sativa, Berberis Vulgaris, Carduus Marinanus, Chelidonium, Grindelia, Passiflora, Pareira, Urtica Urens, Valeriana, etc. are indispensable in these cases; and so, the homoeopath should not allow prejudice against low potencies to mislead. It is recommended that the constitutional remedy be maintained and other low dose remedies be prescribed for acute urgencies which will act sooner than the deep acting constitutional remedy. Some remedies cannot be repeated often like Lycopodium or Sulphur, as constitutional prescriptions, so use of a lower potency, such as 30c may allow the repetition. We may advise the patient to take it 2-3 times a day, but if it is a higher potency like 200c, it is recommended that the remedy given less frequently, plus placebo be given several times in the same day, so that the patient will have psychological satisfaction. We must consider the acute drug for emergency problems, but always a related drug as a constitutional remedy. eq:- Ars, Acon., Bell.

A word of warning in dealing with HIV patients is that their systems must normally be dealt with gently, and so, the prescription of the homoeopathic remedy must be based on rational methods. There is little room for theorizing here. We all tend to be in too much of a hurry, or wish to try a new method discussed in a recent journal or seminar. It is all too often that the homoeopath may misrepresent a symptom that is mentioned in passing, dressing it up to make it a key symptom integral to the case, and focussing the case in a desired direction. The compulsion to use quick or recent methods can

Homoeopathy

easily develop into a compulsion to reach the goal using incorrect symptoms. We all tend to work too quickly on the basis of keynotes, or misrepresenting the importance of dreams or delusions. These methods, while interesting, will not bring the patient's satisfaction. The patient's health is more important than the education of the homoeopath.

It may often be the case that the patient will come to the homoeopath out of desperation, in their final days. The homoeopath can rarely work miracles at this time, and if possible, the homoeopath should attempt to increase the quality of life at this time, by decreasing pains and increasing mental stability. The homoeopath should have a solid knowledge of remedies that can reduce the suffering; acute or specific remedies may be of top priority here. The objective is to delay progression.

9.4 Potency

For a lasting and gentle cure, it is important to adapt the potency to the individual. The terms 'low', medium', and 'high' do not refer to absolute values, and at times a low potency like 30C may, in fact, be too high for the given case. The standard to be used is the reactivity of the diseased organism. Being a special form of regulatory therapy, homoeopathy calls for individualization in determining both the nature and the power of the stimulus. The toxicology based on material doses and the subtle toxicology of homoeopathic drug tests on healthy subjects shows a corresponding affinity of medicinal agents to the level of the disorder: organic lesions can call for low potencies, functional and deep seated disease as well as predominantly mental states may require medium to high potencies. The bio-availability of a drug depends on the method of preparation. The pharmaceutical methods used in homoeopathy 'activate medicinal properties that had previously lay hidden. The lowest effective potency for agents which have no medicinal properties in the crude state is at the level of colloidal solubility (8X). Highly toxic materials should never be given to HIV individuals in low potency.

The fact that individuals living with HIV/AIDS differ greatly in reactive potential, means that the choice of potency has to be adapted to this. Higher potencies, such as 200C should never be given to patients in a parlous state. The more comprehensive the agreement between the disease picture and drug picture, covering also the broad-based constitutional and mental state, the higher the potency selected.

■ ■

Chapter 10

MIASMS

> *The following does not attempt to deliver a biomedical explanation of the development of HIV to AIDS, rather is an attempt to explain the development of HIV to AIDS from a theoretical homoeopathic point of view. An apology must be made for the list of remedies; it is, of course, suggestive; more often to be wholly disregarded. I have followed the lines of earlier homoeopaths in this regard, and given what was then considered the miasmatic remedy, to which I have added my own experience and that of observing practitioners. It is, something to start with at least.*

10.1 Theory

The concept of miasms was originated by Hahnemann before the advent of microbiological tools such as the microscope. It is arguable, that Hahnemann attempted to classify disease according to their microbiological properties.

"Genuine natural chronic diseases have come about through a chronic miasm. Left to themselves and without drug therapy directed specifically against them, they continue to increase, getting worse even if mental and physical dietary regimes are

at their best, with the sufferings the individual undergoes increasing all the time, to the end of his life. Apart from those due to medical mismanagement these are the commonest and most serious tormentors of the human race, for the robustest of constitutions, the best regulated mode of life and most active of vital energies are unable to eradicate them. In conjunction with a mode of life beneficial to body, soul, and spirit, they often go unrecognized for several years in young men during the best years of their youth and in girls whose menstrual cycles are regular in the early stages; those affected appear perfectly healthy to friends and relatives, as though the illness which through infection and hereditary has profoundly marked them had completely vanished, in later years however, it will inevitably reappear when untoward events or conditions pertain in life. It will then increase all the faster and be much more severe in character, the more the vital principle has been put in disarray by destructive passions, grief and worry, and above all, by inappropriate medical treatment.[xcix]

It is, of course, important not to take Hahnemann's concept of miasm too far and call everything that causes illness a miasm. With regards to the often theorized possibility of an HIV or AIDS miasm, this is unlikely as we are looking for the dyscrasia and susceptibilities of our individual constitutions, not of the disease. Let us look at Carcinosinum theory. If a person develops a carcinoma, we cannot treat it as a miasm as it is a single disease and a single drug. Carcinoma is a growth, of two types, benign or malignant; if it is benign then it is psoric or sycotic, but if malignant, then it is tubercular or syphilitic. The miasms are changing as the state of disease changes. So when the person comes to you in HIV infection, you must decide in which stage of the disease they are in. When a person gets infected and he/she comes to us, at that time he/she will likely have a psoric miasm (anxiety), but as soon as this person develops a pathological state, we see the degradation to the syphilitic miasm. The majority of the time of illness is spent in the sycotic and tubercular miasms (induration of glands, pulmonary complaints). The mental symptoms also correspond; they struggle convincing themselves that they can be cured (psora), they try hiding the facts (sycotic), the hatred and blaming of self (syph). Tuberculinum is the most commonly indicated intercurrent remedy in such cases (desire to escape).

10.2 Understanding the Miasmatic Picture: Dominant and Fundamental Miasms

Of the four miasms that are examined, the patient will generally present with a dominant miasm, that is, the picture of the miasm which their disease state is presently in. When the patient reports to the homoeopath, the miasm which is active at the moment is known as the "*Dominant miasm*". The patient may have all miasms present, but at any one time only one miasm is most active or in rarer cases two miasms are very active. The "*Fundamental miasm*", is decided on the basis of the past history and family history of the patient. It gives a clear idea of what the past and what the future course of the disease may be.

Psora: Fundamentally psora is a very healthy sign, it suggests that the person may be brought to health relatively quickly and only requires infrequent treatment constitutionally.

Sycosis: If the sycotic expressions are the base of the patient's health, we may expect a lengthy period of treatment with frequent constitutional treatment.

Tubercular: If the patient has a strong influence of familial

T.B. It may be projected that the patient has a weak base and has to be managed carefully.

Sycotic: If the patient has a history or familial history of syphilis, it is likely that the case will take much time to stabilize to health.

Mixed: If their is a picture of mixed fundamental miasms, the case may be difficult to manage.[2]

10.3 Dominant Miasms

Stage I : (Psora) (Disordered Vata)

It has been mentioned by Dr. Singh that the miasmatic state of the HIV+ individual is normally in a psoric state upon discovery of their situation, although many would argue that this point may also be an acute miasmatic stage, normally due to shock. The shock, which is rational, can explain the dazed appearance, and gradual depression that are observed in the first few weeks after diagnosis. The psoric image is well represented as the patient must struggle to come to terms with this potential threat. There is a denial element often followed by a sense of hope that they will be cured, that the disease will be eradicated from the body; but are often left mentally and emotionally fatigued in a short time. The patient may theorize about the disease or their role in the disease, but this is not practical. The patient may begin or heighten an interest in religion. The anxieties and fears in the early stages are rational and characteristic of this miasm, that is, fear of being alone, of being shunned and not accepted, fear of the illness, fear of death. The patients often become angry, and yet these fits of anger are due to frustration and not directed at anyone, this often alternates with a tearful mood. The patient may wish to be surrounded by loved ones, they tend to suffer from silent grief at this point. The patient may become hypersensitive to impressions of others. It is often at this time that the anger begins, and we see the sycotic state beginning as the patient contemplates evil things, but moreover begins directing the anger at himself. The nervous system is most often affected during this miasm, and will often secondarily affect other systems. Note that the liver may be affected as well as the skin. Ailments at this point are often nervous system related, or due to deficiency. The patient may be mentally very active and wish to be involved in the treatment best suited to him, but will often become tired. It is largely during this stage that the patient can be said to be healthy. Ailments can often be treated simply and are easily eradicated. The body is still quite vital, and the physician should wish to keep the patient in this healthy mode. The ailments are nerve related and we may see the patient having nervous headaches, or indigestion due to nervousness. The skin is often affected and appears unhealthy and dry, possibly with a fungal infection. This should be treated with the correctly chosen internal remedy, as we cannot risk advancing the miasmatic state. The patient may complain of symptoms that are worse in the morning (note the opposite;, syphilis, is worse at night, whilst sycosis is worse in daytime) and is often better during the day, or in the sun. Functional disturbances occur, but often pass, such as constipation, or blocked nose, or dryness of eyes. The physician must prescribe an adequate diet during this stage so as to prevent the lack of or overdose of nutrients in the body. The many symptoms of this stage are related to the anxiety and nervousness, as the patient questions every new ailment or symptom. The appetite is normally decent at this stage and the patient will often manifest cravings, such as for sweets, or hot foods; there may be an aversion to cold foods. Nausea may be present as the patient is over-anxious or he may overeat, for these same reasons diarrhoea may be present. Burning sensation in ailments are normally psoric indications. This stage often develops into more serious pathology as the sycotic state becomes more obvious. If psora is active, a high potency and infrequent repetition is required.

10.4 Remedies to be considered in the psoric state:

Abrotanum, Aconitum, Alumina, Ambra grisea, Ammonium Carbonicum, Anacardium, Antimonium Crudum, Antimonium Tartaricum, Apis Mellifica, Argentum Metallicum, Argentum Nitricum, Arnica Montana, Arsenicum Album , Arsenicum Iodatum , Aurum Metallicum, Baryta Carbonica, Benzoic Acid, Belladonna, Berberis Vulgaris, Borax, Bovista, Bromium, Bufo Rana, Calcarea Arsenicosa, Calcarea Carbonica , Calcarea Iodata, Calcarea Phosphorica, Calcarea Sulphurica, Carbo Animinalis, Carbo Vegetabalis, Capsicum, Causticum, , Chamomilla, Cinabaris, Cistus, Clematis, Coccus Cacti, Colchium, Colocythis, Conium, Crotalus Horridus, Cuprum Metallicum, Digitalis, Dulcamara, Elaterium, Ferrum Metallicum, Ferrum Phosphoricum, Fluoric Acid, Graphites , Hepar Sulphur, Iodum , Kali Bich., Kali Brom., Kali Carb., Kali Iod., Kali Phos., Kali Sulph., Kreosotum, Lac Caninum, Lachesis , Ledum, Lycopodium , Magnesia Carb., Magnesia Phos., Mangan Acetatum, Medorrhinum, Mercurius Sol., Mezereum, Muriatic Acid, Naja Tripudans, Natrum Ars., Natrum Carb., Natrum Mur., Natrum Sulph., Nitric Acid, Nux Vomica, Opium, Origenum, Passiflora, Petroleum, Phosphoric Acid, Phosphorus, Phytolacca, Picric Acid, Platina, Plumbum, Podophyllum, Psorinum , Pulsatilla, Pyrogen, Radium, Ranunculus Bulbosa, Rheum, Rhododendron, Rhus Toxicodendron, Ricinus, Rumex, Ruta, Sabadilla, Sabina, Sambucus, Sanguinaria Canadensus, Sanicula, Sarsaparilla, Secale Cornutum , Selenium , Senicio Aureus, Senega, Sepia, Silicea, Skatol+++, Spigelia, Silicea , Stannum Metallicum, Staphysagaria, Sticta, Stramonium, Sulphur , Sulphuric Acid, Syphilinum, Tabacum, Tarentula Hispanica, Terebinthina, Therideon, Thuja, Tuberculinum , Variolinum, Veratrum Album, Zincum Metallicum.[ci]

Diet : As diet is an important aspect of maintaining health, it is important to follow a regimen that will be regulating and acceptable for the system. For this reason, it is best to follow a diet for the individual constitution and disease. Ayurvedic principles have laid down guidlines to regulate this stage of disease. Foods that are acceptable are:

Grains with butter milk

Chapati, rice

Dal

Lady's finger, French beans, gourd

Apples, figs, papaya, chikoo, custard apple, pineapple

Fruit juices

Spices such as: asafoetida, ginger, black pepper, turmeric, cardamom

Sour items: limes, citrus, tomatoes, tamarind

Cold water

Castor oil, ghee

Avoid :

Fish/ Seafood

Sweets

Mixing food with milk

Idli

Dairy with fruits

Dairy with meats

Dosas

Nuts

Astringent

Avoid eating before meals have been digested

Avoid eating street food

10.6 Stage II: (Sycosis) (Disordered Kapha)

The sycotic stage is often characterized by the self disdain that the patient develops as they become embarrassed and angry at themselves. The patients are suspicious and blame themselves, wonder how this could have happened to them, and why only them. There is often anger and blame directed at those in the immediate environment, and seek attention due to their ailments, often blaming partners who are not infected. The suspicion is misdirected and we will observe the patient often searching for different physicians. There can be a feeling of inferiority, coupled with repentance over past events which can lead to suicide. The patient will dwell upon the sickness. It is at this stage that the dreams and imaginations of the patient are often fixed upon the disease, and we will often hear of the patient complaining of frightful dreams, that is to say, they cannot escape their fear of this disease. The patients often hide away, attempting to conceal their situation from those around them (this is, however, often rational). It might be said that this miasm is often observed in patients who will knowingly infect others, as cruelty is most prevalent here. The patient may exhibit a slowness, of speech, and memory. It should be noted that when sycosis is mixed with psora, this is the basis for the cruel actions; when coupled with syphilis, the basis is explosive or destructive acts to themselves and others. The patients may develop mistrust in themselves and others, resulting in compulsive behaviours such as, pill counting, or recurrent telephone calls to the physician. This miasm produces overgrowth on all aspects, mentally thinking things through again and again; physically in the formation of growths, perhaps as simple as warts, or as serious as hyperplasia and cancers. The organs most often affected are the pelvic organs, and attacks tissues such as endodermal and soft tissues. We may observe premature gray hair or increase in hair growth, nevi on the head, and nevi and condylomata on areas where there is moisture, such as the genitalia. The beginning stages of opacification of the lens of the eye often begins in this state. There tend to be discharges from all orifices, which are often yellow or green; note that the discharge will often ameliorate the local symptoms. The patient may appear pale and lymphatic (diathesis) and may appear to have difficulty catching his/her breath. Pains may be rheumatic and tend to come and go suddenly. The patient may develop a craving for alcohol or drugs, as this is a way of avoiding the situation. At this time we would hope that the appetite remains substantial. The patient may suffer from painful nephritis or renal insufficiency. The patient may suffer severe diarrhoea as peristalsis is accelerated, enuresis may occur. As with all discharges, the stool and urine may be corrosive and painful, causing itching. The perspiration may come on during sleep. The patient is generally better in dry weather and worse in the damp, so an increase in colds can be expected. If sycosis is active, a low or medium potency and frequent repetition is required.

10.7 Remedies to be considered

> Abrotanum, Actae Racemosa, Agaricus Muscarus, Alumina, Ammonium Carbonicum, Anacardium, Antimonium Crudum, Antimonium Tartaricum, Apis Mellifica, Argentum Metallicum, Argentum Nitricum, Arsenicum Album, Arsenicum Iodatum, Aurum Metallicum, Baryta Carbonica, Benzoic Acid, Berberis Vulgaris, Borax, Bovista, Bufo Rana, Calcarea Arsenicosa, Calcarea Carbonica, Calcarea Iodatum, Calcarea Phosphorica, Calcarea Sulphurica, Carbo Animalis, Carbo Vegatabalis, Capsicum, Causticum, Chamomila, Cinnaberis, Coccus Cacti, Colchium, Conium, Crotalus Horridus, Digitalis, Dulcamara, Ferrum Mettalicum, Fluoric Acid, Graphites, Hepar Sulphur Calcarea, Iodium, Kali Bichromicum, Kali Bromatum, Kali Carbonicum, Kali Iodatum, Kali Sulphuricum, Kreosotum, Lac Canninum, Lachesis, Ledum, Lycopodium, Magnesia Carbonica, Magnesia Muriatica, Medhorrhinum, Mercurius Corrosivus, Mercurius Solubilus, Mezereum, Naja Tripudans, Natrum Arsenicum, Natrum Carbonicum, Natrum Muriaticum,

Natrum Sulph, Nitric Acid, Nux Vomica, Opium, Petroleum, Phosphorus, Phytolacca, Picric Acid, Platina, Plumbum, Podophylum, Psorinum, Pulsatilla, Pyrogenum , Radium , Ranunculus Bulbosus, Rhododendron, Rhus Toxicodendron, Ruta, Sanguinarius Canadensus, Sanicula, Sarsaparilla , Secal Cornutum, Selenium, Senicio Aureus, Sepia , Silicea , Stannum Metallicum, Staphysagria, Sticta, Stramonium, Sulphur, Syphilinum, Tabacum, Tarentula Hispanica, Terebinthina, Thuja, Tuberculinum, Variolinum, Veratrum Album, Zincum Metallicum.[cii]

Diet:

Cereals

Roasted pulses (dal)

Juicy fruits

Egg white

Vegetables that hold water

Chapati

Jaggery

Leafy vegetables

Bitter gourd

Spices: turmeric, fenugreek, cumin, nutmeg, saffron, cardamom, coriander

Avoid:

Seafood

Sour

Salty

Sweetmeats

Excessively sweet things

Basmati rice

Bhakris

Phulkas

Avoid eating before previous meal is digested

Avoid eating street food

10.9 Stage III: (Tubercular) (Disordered Vata Kapha)

The remedy Tuberculinum is said to be the most often prescribed intercurrent remedy. The tubercular miasm is perhaps most often present over the extended period of time as the patient gradually declines in health. The tubercular miasm is easily observed in the patient as they become increasingly apathetic to their own situation. They are often not tolerant of the health regimen with which they should adhere to and will often purposely avoid it. This miasm is characterized by changeability, and the patient will change diet, physician, friends, and outlook. The patients care for nothing, even themselves or their ailments, and will often not accept advice in regard to health and food. They become irritated, fearful, and disgusted with themselves. It is at an extreme point in this miasm in which the patient will become weak and fatigued, loss of weight and wasting occurs (slimming). It is in the tubercular stage that one can observe the characteristic AIDS Related Complex (ARC) The scrofulous diathesis may be observed (generalized lymphadenopathy, and hardening of the glands). This stage is characterized by depletion, drainage, and wasting; often due to glandular changes. Anemia and immune mediated thrombocytopaenia are often discovered. The latter stages of this miasm may appear in serious lifethreatening ailments such as meningitis; pains so much that they must knock their heads against objects, or cover the head. Blindness may occur at the later stages, along with streptococcal infections of the eustachian tube. This miasm may allow disease that has long passed to reappear: shingles, herpes, etc. Intense fevers may be observed, often during the night, which can be accompanied by haemorrhages, such as epistaxis, or blocked orifices such as the nose or rectum. The mouth is often affected by thrush, accompanied by albuminous or blood stained ulcers. This miasm is chiefly to blame for the occurrence of serious respiratory infections. Pneumonia, pneumo carinii, tuberculosis, bronchitis, COPD, often begin during the tubercular state, and will extend into syphilitic as the patient's health declines. The lymphatics of the abdomen, aswell as mesenteric glands are often hardened or swollen. The characteristic diarrhoea can often be observed, and is often accompanied by blood. Renal insufficiency may be observed. The skin symptoms are progressively worsened during this miasm and what may begin as a fungal growth may develop into bedsores, or severe boils. It should be noted that these skin ailments should not be suppressed as the patient often develops respiratory complications. The patient may begin to be fatigued, mentally and physically, progressing to a state of exhaustion, never seems to get rest. Tired at night and also after sleep. Blood results should be particularly noted during any point in the tubercular miasm, and consultation with experts at any necessary time is of utmost importance. We will often see this miasm followed by the syphilitic miasm.

If the tubercular miasm is active one must be very careful in selecting potency and repetition. If you give too high a potency and repetition is frequent it may produce an aggravation. With regards to prescribing the nosodes, there are two distinct opinions: the first would suggest beginning with repeated dosages of the tuberculinum nosode, or bacillinum if there are prominent skin symptoms, until a mild drug proving occurs, followed by the indicated constitutional drug; the second opinion believes that this method would severely disrupt the case and so a moderate potency of the nosode as an intercurrent remedy is more gently tolerated. The reasoning behind developing a drug proving in the immunecompromized individual is to rouse the system. However, lower potencies of indicated or miasmatic drugs will similarly build up the constitution over time. Arsenicum Iodatum, in very low potency over time is said to improve the patient's constitution. Ars. iod. has proved a picture most closely related of any remedy to the miasm and phthisis.

10.10 Remedies to be considered in the tubercular stage

> Abrotanum, Agaricus Muscarus, Alfalfa+++Ammonium Carb., Anacardium+++, Argentum Nitricum, Arsenicum Album+++, Arsenicum Iodatum, Aurum Metallicum, Baryta Carbonica, Benzoic Acid, Belladonna, Bromium, Bufo Rana, Calcarea Arsenicosa, Calcarea Carbonica, Calcarea Phosphorica , Calcarea Sulphurica, Calendula, Carbo Animalis, Carbo Vegetabalis, Causticum, Chamomilla, Conium, Crotalus Horridus, Dulcamara, Ferrum Metallicum, Ferrum Phosphoricum, Fluoric Acid, Graphites, Hepar Sulphur, Hydrastis Canadensus+++, Hydrocotyle , Iodum, Kali Bichromicum, Kali Carbonicum, Kali Iodatum, Kali Phosphoricum, Kali Sulphuricum, Kreosotum, Lac Caninum, Lachesis, Lycopodium, Magnesia Carbonica, Magnesia Muriatica, Muriatic Acid, Naja Tripudans, Natrum Muriaticum+++, Natrum Sulphuricum, Nitric Acidic, Phosphoric Acid, Phosphorus, Phytolacca, Psorinum, Pyrogen, Radium, Rumex, Sabadilla, Sanguinara Canadensus, Sarsaparilla, Selenium, Senecio Aureus, Senega, Sepia, Silicea, Spigelia, Spongia, Stannum Metallicum, Sticta, Stramonium, Sulphur, Sulphuric Acid, Syphilinum, Tarentula, Terebinthina, Teucrium+++,Theridion, Thuja, Tuberculinum, Zincum Metallicum.[ciii]

10.11 Diet

Lime

Tomato

Citrus fruits

Papaya

Pepper

Vegetables

Supplements

Milk with ginger powder

Ghee

Cauliflower

Leafy vegetables

Cabbage

Pumpkin

Sweet potato

Radish

Avoid:

Sea food

Spicy

Caffeine

Alcohol

Overeating

Pungent food

Sour food

Salty food

Avoid eating before previous meal has been digested.

Avoid eating street food.

10.12 Stage IV: (Syphilitic) (Disordered Pitta)

Many knowledgeable physicians would suggest that it is most likely the syphilitic stage at which the patient simultaneously develops AIDS. Previous to this, in the psoric, sycotic, and tubercular miasms, there has been a degradation of health and increased susceptibility to disease (opportunistic infections). This can also be noticed on the mental plane as the patient becomes increasingly disillusioned with his/her treatment and the likelihood of success. The patient is often melancholic and attempts to ready himself for death. There is a characteristic desire for solitude, which can be a risk factor for suicide. It is at this point where the patients become destructive to themselves, they no longer have sympathy or affection for anything, and rage often abounds. It is likely that at this point dementia may occur. There is often intense pain as the system begins to be degraded. The patient may be unable to realize the pain. The patient is restless, but intensely fatigued and sleep is often difficult. The appetite is lost. Physically there is destruction and perversion of the tissues, particularly the mesodermal tissues, soft tissue and bone; glandular tissues previously enlarged are now degraded. The patient is most often emaciated as there is destruction of tissues and loss of the body to assimilate proper materials from foods. Aphtous ulceration can be seen in the soft palate, along with the overgrowth of yeast (oral thrush). There is often a loss of control of both rectum and urinary organs, often accompanied by a foul odor. There are perversions in the blood stream and the often misunderstood Kaposi's sarcoma may fungate or penetrate soft tissue, and invade bone; later disseminating into lymphnodes. Dysplasias are common. Serious complications occur in the CNS, and meningitis, encephalitis, septicemia may occur. The condition at this point is often associated with neuropathies and sensory loss. If this miasm is dominant you need to prescribe a low to medium potency with minimum repetition if possible. If it is the beginning of the syphilitic stage you need to prescribe in medium or high potency, so as to prevent further progression of the disease.

10.13 List of anti- syphilitic remedies to consider:

Obviously not all remedies were considered and those mentioned can be argued, however, these remedies have proven themselves most efficacious in the treatment of the miasm. The leading remedies are highlighted.

Acetic Acid, Alfalfa ,Anacardium, Antimonium Chlor., Apis, Arsenicum Album, Arsenicum Iodatum, Aurum Metallicum , Baryta Carb., Benzoic Acid, Calc. Ac., Calc. Ars., Calc. Carb., Calc. Iod., Calc. Sulph., Carbo Anim., Carbo Veg., Causticum, Chamamilla, Cinnabaris, Clematis, Conium, Condurango, Crotalus Horridus, Elateria, Euphorb., Fluoric Acid , Galium, Graphites, Helleborous, Hepar Sulphur, Hydrastis Canadensus+++, Iodum, Kali Bich , Kali Carb., Kali Iod, Kali Sulph, Kreosotum, Lachesis , Ledum, Lycopodium, Medhorrinum, Merc Cor., Merc Sol., Mezereum, Nat. Mur., Nat. Sul., Nitric Acid , Opium, Pareira, Passiflora, Phos Acid, Phos, Phytolacca , Psorinum, Pyrogen, Radium, Ratania, Sarsaparilla, Selenium, Sepia, Silicea, Stannum Met., Staph, Stramonium, Sulph., Sulphuric Acid, Syphilinum, Terebinthenum+++, Thuja, Tuberculinum.[civ]

10.14 Combination Therapy:

For many homoeopaths the notion of using combination of remedies is unthinkable and closely linked to a sacrilegious activity. However, homoeopathy is a science, not a cult, and so, deviating against the path is not a sin, rather simply questionable. Questions require answers, so before the notion is condemned, let us examine the methods used, and more importantly, the results. Often homoeopathic combinations act as allopathic remedies would, with similar results, the short lived amelioration of symptoms. The main argument against combinations is that it is impossible to know which of the drugs in the combination acted curatively. However, those in favor of combinations argue that this makes no difference, as when the patient appears at the next meeting he/she will be in another disease state anyway.

The combination remedies that have been developed for the treatment of HIV are based on the theory of prevention and prophylaxis. That is, they are taken regularly enough so that the specific site targeted by the given drug may be stimulated; for example, Aconite, is useful in the earliest stages of all inflammations, therefore, the intended action is to prevent inflammation. One preparation of combination formula that has been used is Acon. 6c, Aur-met 6c, Bapt. 6c, Card.-M., M.T., Cham. 6c, Chel. M.T., Echin. 6c, Ferr.-ph. 6c, Gels. 6c, Gunp. 6c, Kali-ph. 6c, and Nat-m. 6c.

Combination medicines, however, have a greater likelihood in disordering the system and making the symptom picture cloudy. Much more study will have to be made of these remedies before they are administered to ailing patients.

■■

Chapter 11

COST

11.1 Cost

The cost of homoeopathic medicines is negligible in comparison to the expense of the present allopathic and ayurvedic treatments. To purchase one vial of medicine containing 60 impregnated pellets costs 4-7Rs (12-21 cents CAN). It is likely that one to two vials would suffice for a month's worth of medicine. The major cost incurred would be the visit to a homoeopath, which can range from 20Rs to 200Rs (70 cents - $8 CAN).. However, in the majority of townships in India, and certainly Gujarat, a charitable institute can provide treatment free of charge.

11.2 Eradication

It is highly unlikely that a cure presently exists, despite the conspiracy theories of many individuals. However, the demonstration that Highly Active AntiRetroviral Therapy (HAART) can suppress HIV replication below detectable levels does pose the theory that if suppression can exist long enough, the few cells containing the HIV may die or be killed by the host immune system; and hence the patient will be cured. This does sound like a logical possibility; however, time will tell, and it will likely require more advanced chemotherapies. There are anatomical and physiological areas where the virus may remain that may be difficult for drugs to access; the CNS and prostate are possible examples. With regards to cellular changes, it is observed that HIV integrates into chromosomal DNA in presently nonreplicating form, but with the possibility of replicating in future. The reason that large studies in this vein are unavailable is that long term use of HAART results in side effects and so the time required before cellular mortality occurs is presently only theoretical.

Chapter 12

PROPOSAL TO NATIONAL HIV TEAM

12.1 Proposal

The following proposal was presented to the National HIV team of the Salvation Army on September 25/99. A total of twenty- two team members were present. As a result of the presentation, Captain G. has presented the findings to three groups.

Proposal for Integration of Homoeopathic Therapeutics into the Treatment Schedule of HIV patients at the Hospital.

12.2 Objective

To integrate homoeopathy as a viable resource in the treatment of HIV individuals at the Hospital.

12.3 Reason

Recent studies undertaken by the Central Council of Homoeopathy and the Canadian College of Naturopathic Medicine have revealed that homoeopathic medicines can provide an efficient drug regimen to maintain health in asymptomatic HIV carriers. At present, efficient antiretroviral medications and protease inhibitors are largely unavailable to the patients in the region of Anand, due to the high cost. The average cost of a monthly drug regimen of Zidudovine (AZT) is Rs.30,000/-, which is financially impossible for the present PLWHA in Anand as they have a monthly in come of Rs.1000/- on an average. Therefore, the patients at the hospital have been receiving symptomatic treatment for their ailments and no medications are available to maintain health during asymptomatic periods. However, counselling and nutritional advice have been undertaken. Reviews of the literature by the CCH and CCNM reveal that homoeopathy can provide a cost effective health maintenance regime for asymptomatic periods, therefore reducing the number of opportunistic infections and elongating the healthy life of the patients.

12.4 Method

As homoeopathic medicines cost an average of Rs.15/- per month's supply, if purchased from local retailers, it may be possible for the hospital to acquire a large selection for a lower cost, to be distributed by the hospital dispensary. It is also likely possible for a donation to make the purchase of the supply from Homoeopathic pharmacy in Anand, therefore reducing the cost of the medicine to zero for the hospital. As homoeopathic medicines are available in liquid form and liquid impregnated pellet form, it would be wise to purchase all medicines in liquid form along with a substantial amount of blank pellets; to be impregnated when required. This will allow for further cost effective methods as the quantity of medicine used will be substantially reduced.

Proposal to National HIV Team

Volunteer homoeopathic medical students in internship are available for consultation at no charge. The students have received education in both the homoeopathic and allopathic systems of medicine and would be a useful addition to the HIV field unit due to their accessibility and availability. These students are able to make medical diagnosis and could make recommendations for further treatment under the direction of their teachers. The volunteer doctors would be educated in the homoeopathic method of treatment for HIV by the author. The approach to the homoeopathic treatment in HIV is to promote health through nutritional and exercise schedules, aswell as through homoeopathic prescriptions which stimulate the body to maintain homoeostasis. The homoeopathic system of medicine, owes its origin to the German physician Christian Frederick Samuel Hahnemann. The system was introduced by him in The Organon of the Art of Healing in 1810. Homoeopathy has been used widely, with its primary emphasis on therapeutics. Besides treating the immediate disease, it strengthens the body's defense mechanism leading to long term health. In this sense it plays a significant preventative and promotive role in healthcare. Homoeopathy is based upon two major demonstrable principles: the law of similars, and the law of minimum dose.

The law of similars assumes that every symptom is the reaction of the defense mechanism of the human body against the disease causing agents. "The substance that can produce specific symptoms in a healthy human being can cure those same symptoms in a sick individual. Homoeopathy is known for its use of microdoses of the symptom causing substance for cure. The microdose is considered to act as a catalytic agent to further stimulate and strengthen the existing defense mechanism of the body, and thus bring about cure.

The use of the classical approach to homoeopathy, as described above, would require regular visits to patients, approximately bi-weekly. However, it may be possible to introduce a systematic combination of remedies for patients who are not readily accessible. Alternatively, the Homoeopathic Hospital in Anand, offer free out patient clinics six days per week. This option may be preferable to some patients as the doctors attending the clinics have many years of experience; however, this setting would not allow as much time for the patient as would be available from the internship doctors.

12.5 Cost

The total cost of the initial purchase of medicines from homoeopathic pharmacy is Rs.5000/- for approximately 400 different remedies, ample blank pellets, and ample administrative containers. It is likely that this amount of money can be obtained by sponsorship from a foreign source, Allen's Restaurant of Toronto, Canada. Further costs would not be required for some time. The doctors of homoeopathy are volunteering their time and resources, and the Out-Patients Department (OPD's) of the aforementioned hospitals work on a charitable basis, so cost is not incurred for consultation. A negotiable cost may be involved in some cases for the patient, depending on the decision of the hospital administration so that the patient may value the treatment.

12.6 Time Schedule

Should this application be accepted by the hospital administration it is likely that the program could begin within one to two weeks. This time allotment would allow procuring of medicaments and training of the homoeopaths. The homoeopaths would be available, on-call, seven days per week. It would be preferable if the hospital HIV unit would supply the transportation to and from the necessary home visits.

Chapter 13

CONCLUSION

Many microbial diseases have posed a threat to the survival of mankind but none has succeeded in completely eliminating a species higher up in evolution. Small pox has had a devastating effect; cholera has decimated villages; Ricketsiae have destroyed armies and changed the course of history; yet mankind survived. It may be that HIV is in a state of flux and is incessantly endeavouring to find its equilibrium in host parasite relationship. Could it be that nature is trying to redefine the role of immune system in general and the role of CD4 T cells in particular? For after all, some experts do believe that sickle trait in humans in improved by malaria burden[1].

There is no doubt that the major step towards dealing with the spread of HIV is decent public health education, focusing on the eradication of *fear* of the disease. That patients may be accepted and loved, so that they may focus on healing rather than hiding.

Fear is an undeniable source of disease. Could it be that fear and shame are as representative of this disease as weightloss and sweating. It could well be that overcoming this fear and shame are the first steps in eradicating the pandemic.

It has been the findings of many leaders in this field that for a patient to become a long term survivor three things are required:

1) **the will to live-** if the patient feels that they are punished or are the victims of moral blame they will not thrive.

2) **to enjoy life-** if the patient remains thinking about the disease or is self destructive, they will not thrive. Anger and anxiety will eventually manifest as pathology.

3) **they must become actively involved in their health-** the patient must attempt to maintain high levels of hygiene and nutrition, they must be informed[2].

PHOTOGRAPHIC CODOCIL

"In the face of uncertainty there is nothing wrong with hope"

The following photographs represent the situation in rural and urban Inadia. Several photographs were taken by the author, others by professional photographers.

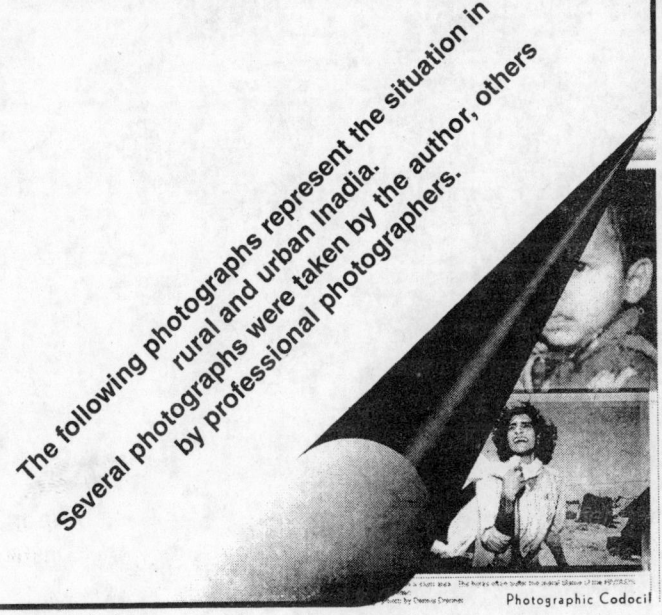

Photographic Codocil

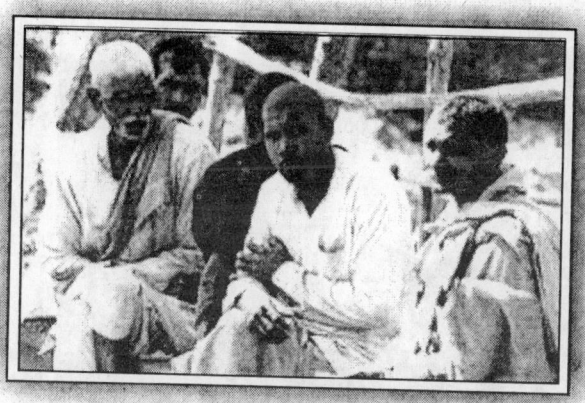

Photo 1.1 : Rural Patients

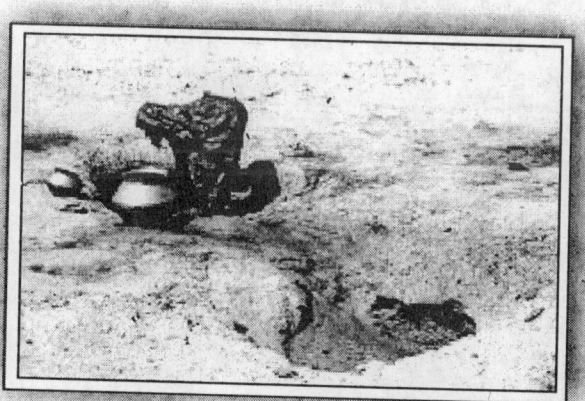

Photo 1.2 : Poor Hygiene and Water

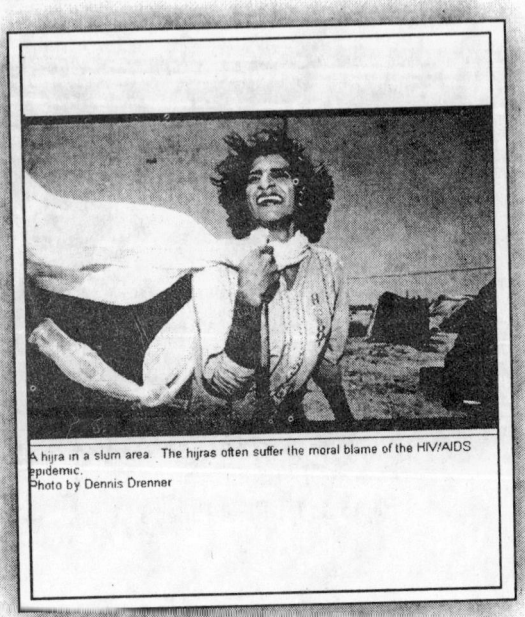

Photo 1.3 : The Hijras, often the victims of moral blame.
Photo *by Dennis Dremmer*

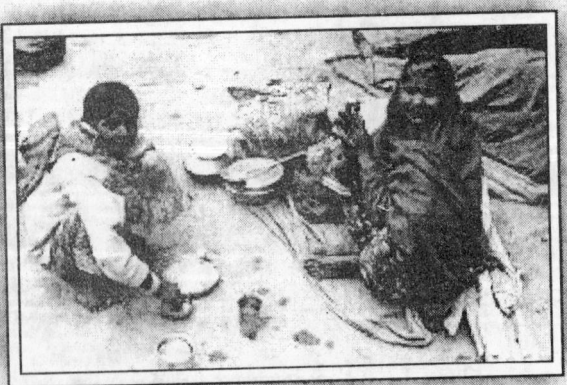

Photo 1.4 : Poor Hygiene and Nutrition

Photographic Codocil

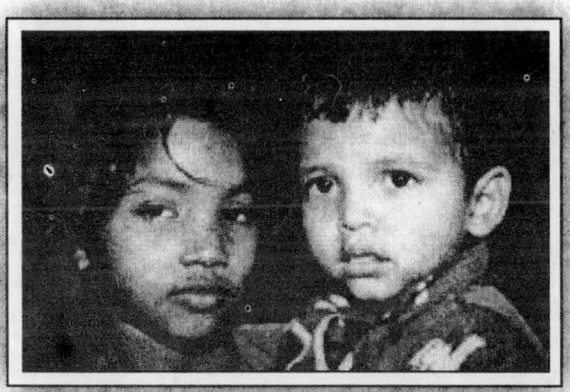

Photo 1.5 : Young Children Must Often Raise Themselves

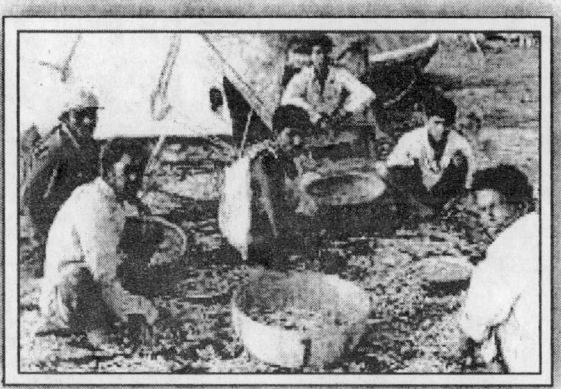

Photo 1.6 : Rural Slum Setting

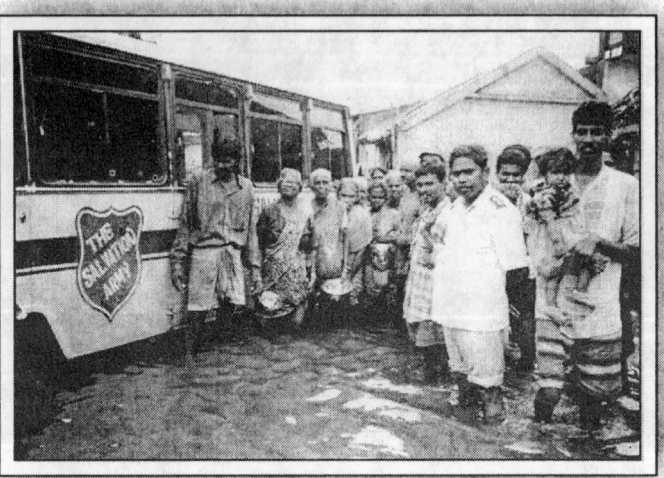

Photo 1.7 : Continual Hardships & Disease Sources

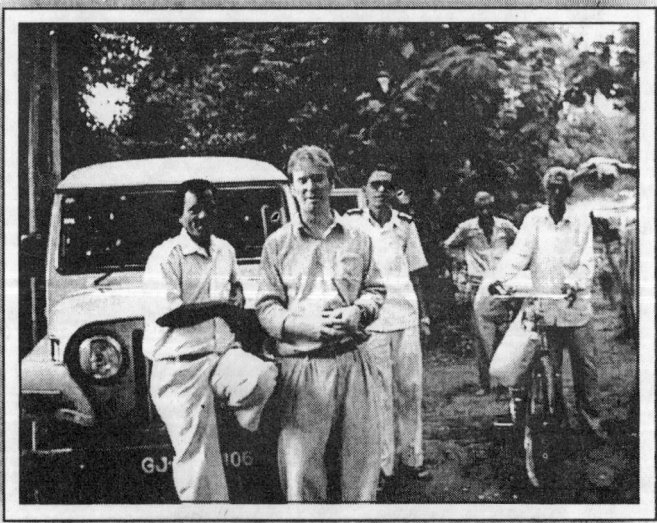

Photo 1.8 : Author with Emery Field Team in Rural Jungle Area

Photographic Codocil

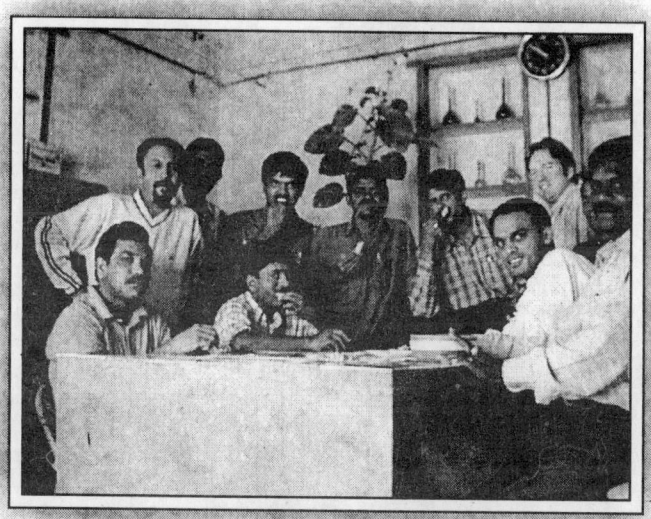

Photo 1.9 : Emery Hospital HIV Team in Lab

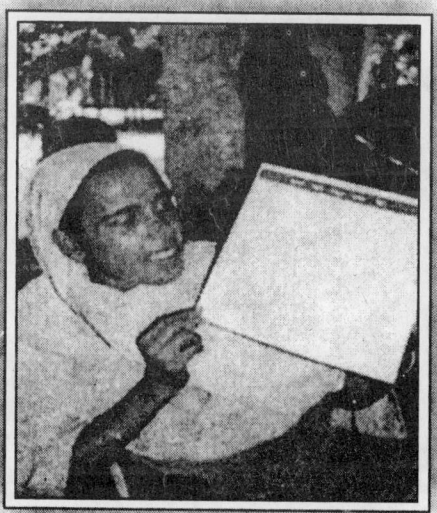

Photo 2.1 : Local Empowerment. Women Teach Women.

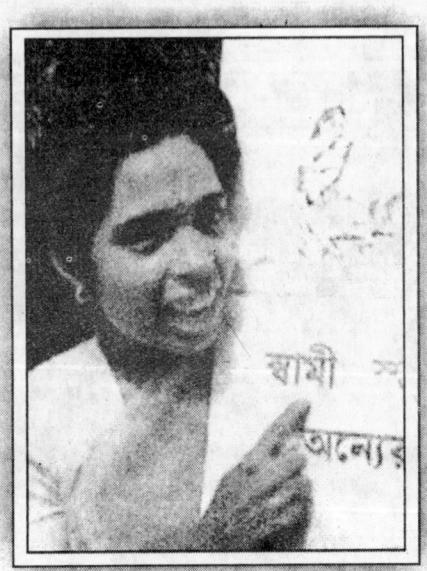

Photo 2.2 : Sexual Education by Concerned Women's Groups

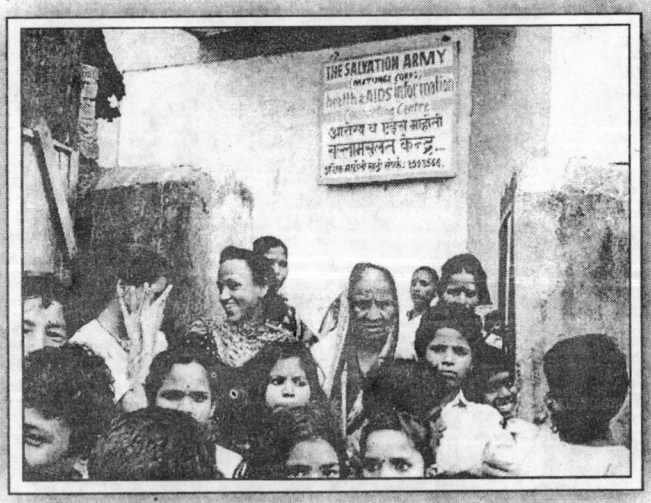

Photo 2.3 : Mumbai HIV/AIDS Clinic.

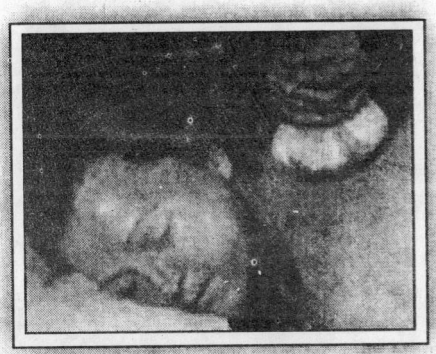

Photo 3.1 : Ayurvedic Panchakarma.[2]

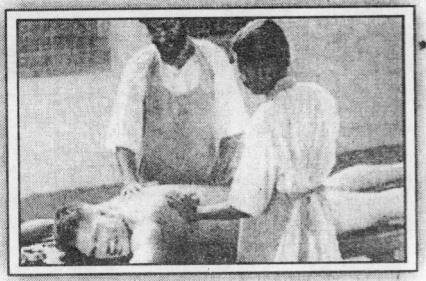

Photo 3.2 : Ayurvedic Panchakarma

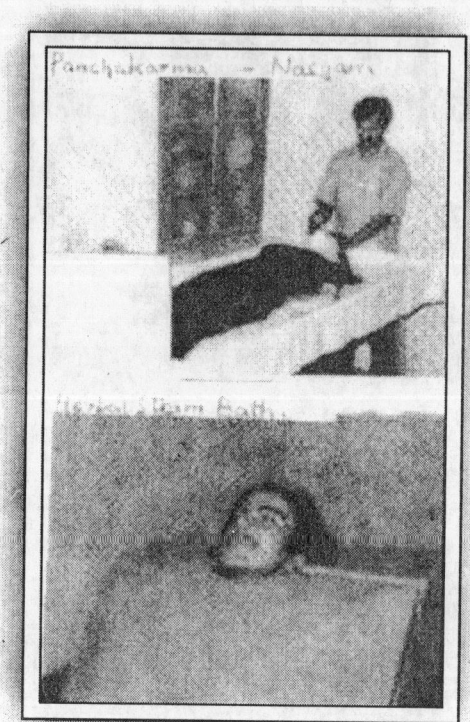

3

Photo 3.4 : Ayurvedic Panchakarma Hot Oil Treatment and Steam Treatment[4]

---

[2] Phota Copyright of Sukhada Hospital, Kochi, Kerala, India
[3] ibid
[4] Photo Copyright of M/S Sukhodaya Ayurvedic Hospital, Kottayam, Kerala, India.

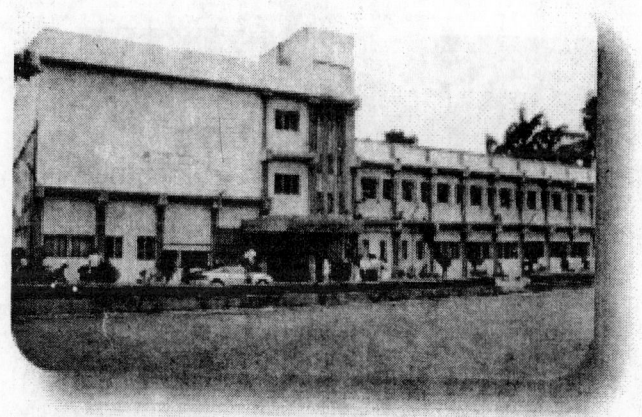

Photo 4.1 : C.M.P. Homoeopathic College[5]

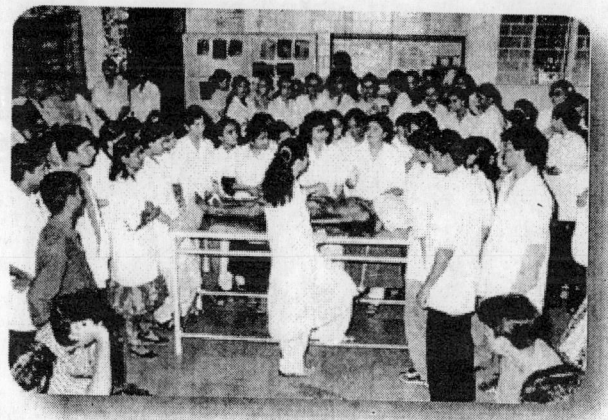

Photo 4.2 : C.M.P. Hom. College Lectures[6]

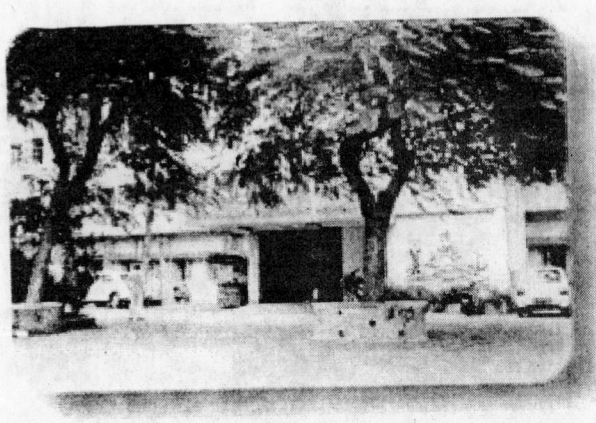

Photo 4.3: Shree Mumbadevi Homoeopathic Hospital[7]

---

[5] Phota Courtesy of CMP Homoeopathic Medical College, HES, Irla Naka, Mumbai, India
[6] Ibid
[7] Ibid

Annexure

CASE STUDY

Original Research and Audit:

A Pilot Retrospective Case Control Study on the Efficacy of Homoeopathic Treatment in Rural Indian HIV Carriers

E.J.MILLS[1], S.J. CHRISTIAN[2], K. JAIN[3], T. JAIN[4], C.ROSS[5]

Abstract:

To assess the role of homoeopathic medicines in the treatment of late stage HIV infection, a pilot study was conducted by the above mentioned in India starting in August 1999. 40 late stage HIV carriers (28 male and 12 female) were randomly selected from case histories. 20 individuals had received no antiretroviral or immunotherapy medications, but were treated symptomatically by the standard allopathic medicines. The remaining 20 individuals were treated homoeopathically using potencies varying from 30 CH to CM, and in varying dosage and medicine, depending on the age and constitution of the individual patients. Some patients in the latter group also received symptomatic allopathic treatment. All but four of the group receiving only allopathic treatment deteriorated in health, and/or subsequently died. All but two of the patients receiving homoeopathic treatment remained healthy. Efforts should be made to determine haematological and immunological status.

KEYWORDS : Homoeopathy; HIV infection; AIDS; ARC.

1. Public Health Officer, Homoeopathic Researcher
2. Emery Hospital HIV Unit Coordinator, Research Assistant
3. Homoeopathic Physician, Research Assistant
4. Allopathic Physician, Research Assistant
5. Vice President Academic, Program Director Public Health Dept., Canadian College of Naturopathic Medicine.

Correspondence: E.J. Mills, Canadian College of Naturopathic Medicine, 1255 Shepherd Avenue East, North York, Ontario, Canada, M2K1E2

Introduction:

Acquired ImmunoDeficiency Syndrome (AIDS) refers to the occurrence of a life threatening opportunistic infection which may otherwise be dealt with swiftly by the body's natural protective measures (immune system). AIDS is common in India as the majority of Human ImmunoDeficiency Virus (HIV) carriers are unaware until late stage HIV, when AIDS Related Complex (ARC) or opportunistic infections have compromised the immune system. The stage for AIDS is set by the HIV, a retrovirus which infects the lymphocytes, particularly those with CD4 receptors, and later monocytes, macrophages, and B- cells. The aforementioned cells are primarily responsible for the immune capabilities of the individual. The HIV infection, which is certainly tragic, may not be fatal. However, opportunistic infections and cancerous growths, which do not respond to the normal treatment in late stage HIV carriers, almost always prove fatal. Evidence now shows that HIV infection, whilst chronic in nature, may allow the individual to live anywhere from 2 years to indefinitely. However, as successful anti-viral and protease inhibitors drugs are largely unavailable in third world countries, the life span of an individual infected with HIV can average far lower, depending on previous health, mental state, hygiene, nutrition, and exercise. To date, conventional drugs do not cure an individual of HIV, however, research continues.

A number of vaccine trials have been undertaken and newer studies look promising. However, we must consider the complex make up of the HIV and the frequency with which it changes structure. We must also consider that presently HIV 1 and HIV 2 can be blamed for the pandemic. Unfortunately, financial constraints have somewhat effected studies for the benefit of the third world and one could reasonably contest that the pharmaceutical world is overlooking its charitable duties. Concerted efforts must be made by all medical personnel to some extent to evolve effective treatment for this disease, which can potentially effect the world's population. Decent public health education has been the most successful method of prevention to date. However, as the emphasis on HIV is declining, through health trends, an increase in HIV infection can be expected in developed countries throughout the world. Due to lack of public health education in third world countries, often related to low literacy rates, the rate of infection has seen a consistent growth since HIV was first discovered. HIV therapies focusing on the symptomatic phase of HIV/AIDS must be all the more necessary as the rate of world wide infection soars. If these infections are not cured or treated successfully, they will add to the global socio- ecological and cultural devastation that is presently being witnessed, as seen in Sub-Saharan Africa.

The homoeopathic system of medicine, used in group Y, owes its origin to the German physician Christian Frederick Samuel Hahnemann. The system was introduced in his famous writings entitled "The Organon of Rational Medical Practice" in 1810. Homoeopathy has been used widely, with its primary emphasis on therapeutics. Besides treating the immediate disease, it strengthens the body's defense mechanism leading to long term health. In this sense it plays a significant preventative and promotive role in healthcare. Homoeopathy is based upon two major demonstrable principles: the law of similars, and the law of minimum dose.

The law of similars assumes that every symptom is the reaction of the defense mechanism of the human body against the disease causing agents. The substance that can produce specific symptoms in a healthy human being can cure those same symptoms in a sick individual. Homoeopathy is known for its use of microdocos of the symptom causing substance for cure. The microdose is considered to act as a catalytic agent to further stimulate and strengthen the existing defense mechanism of the body, and thus bring about cure.

Homoeopathic medicines have been found effective in viral infections, such as meningitis, influenza, pertussis, etc. Homoeopathic medicines have also proven useful as prophylaxis against epidemics, however, this is unlikely in the case of HIV. Therapeutic efficacy in retroviral infection is, to date, largely unavailable and has yet to be evaluated on a grand scale. It may be argued that homoeopathy has not played a large published role in the treatment of retroviral infections as discovery of a retrovirus was only made in 1980 when the human T-cell lymphotrophic virus (HTLV-1) was linked to T-cell leukemia. A number of studies on homoeopathic treatments in HIV have been published and the results are, at times, questionable. Therefore, it has been of utmost importance in our study to maintain a consistent protocol. Continued organized research is required to reveal if homoeopathy may be a viable therapy, and possible alternative to antiretroviral drugs; particularly for those who the modern drugs are a financial impossibility. It was therefore necessary, for the above mentioned individuals to conduct a study, to ascertain the role of homoeopathic medicines in the treatment of late stage HIV infection.

Table 1.1 : Participants in study, age and sex distribution:

(n= 40)

Age Groups (in years)	Total	X-male	X-female	Y-male	Y-female
1 day to 5years	0	0	0	0	0
6-15	2	0	0	2	0
16-25	4	1	2	1	0
26-35	20	7	2	6	5
36-45	11	5	2	4	0
46-55	2	0	0	2	0
56 and above	1	1	0	0	0
Total *(n)*	**40**	**14**	**6**	**15**	**5**

Table 1.2 : Mode of infection relative to participants.

Mode of Infection	Total	X-male	X-female	Y-male	Y-female
Sexual Contact					
-heterosexual:	20	10	4	6	0
-homosexual :	0	0	0	0	0
(commercial sex workers):	1	0	1	0	0
(commercial sex users):	11	6	0	5	0
Contaminated Blood/Blood Products:	15	2	2	6	5
Infected Needles:	0	0	0	0	0
Materno- foetal	1	0	0	1	0
Undetermined:	4	2	0	2	0

MATERIALS and METHODS

A total of 40 individuals of varying stages of HIV infection were randomly selected according to availability of resources. All of the 40 patients represent similar educational and financial backgrounds, that is, largely uneducated and invariably poor with an income rarely exceeding 1000Rs ($35 CAN) per month. The majority of patients had been tested positive as a result of common ailments not responding to conventional treatments, for example, tuberculosis, fever, diarrhoea, etc. Screening of the X group was done by Sero-Strip or Tri-Dot at the Salvation Army Emery Hospital in Anand, Gujarat. To rule out false positives, the results were confirmed by the standard Western Blot. Due to the high costs of CD4+ level testing, few individuals have been tested. The method of determining health status is through the diagnosis of attending physicians.

Case Study

The testing of the X group patients was performed at the Emery Hospital laboratory under the direction of Mr. & Mrs. S. Christian. Presently the Tri- Dot method is employed as this method is most-effective and takes only seconds. A positive Tri- Dot test must be confirmed by a Western Blot test. The Western Blot test is quite expensive (2000Rs, $70CAN) and so, samples for testing are normally sent to the government laboratories of the National AIDS Research Institute (NARI) in Pune, Maharashtra.

The patients case histories were examined or the patients were interviewed to ascertain the probable time and mode of infection. A number of the patients from X group had deceased or expired during the research, however, their histories can continue to be used as reasonable example of patients not receiving immune system treatment, as their deterioration in health was typical. These patients received no antiretroviral treatment or protease inhibitors due to lack of availability in India and the subsequent cost of those available. At present the antiretroviral drugs Zidovudine (AZT) and Dideoxyinosine (DDI) are extremely costly and largely unaffordable to the patients, the cost is on an average 30,000Rs ($1050 CAN) per month, impossible for the patients earning a measly 1000Rs ($35 CAN) per month when healthy. All of the patients in group X received allopathic treatment symptomatically; this included the various Anti Koch Treatment (AKT) combinations for tuberculosis, paracetamol analgesics, Acyclovir for herpes zoster related eruptions, Metronazole ointment and Nystatin for oral and vaginal thrush, etc. X group did, however, receive occasional counselling and visits from the HIV Field team of the Emery Hospital. The patients were recommended to maintain a proteinous diet, with foods easily digestible. However, few of the X group can be said to have been actively involved in their health, through exercise or seeking spiritual resources.

The majority simply relied upon the staff of the Field Team. The patients represent the majority of HIV infected individuals of past and present in the Gujarat state as they were invariably poor and uneducated; the men worked primarily in labour related fields and the women as cleaners.

The Y group were initially diagnosed HIV+ from testing in private and government laboratories, using the ELISA methods. The results were further confirmed by the Western Blot test. Several of the Y group had CD4, CD3, and CD8 counts tested on at least one occassion to determine whether antiretroviral drugs may be of benefit. However, none of the patients from Y group received any antiretroviral treatment, and the majority of treatment has been with homoeopathic medicines under the direction of Drs. K. and T. Jain. The total cost of the homoeopathic medicines is 60Rs ($2.20 CAN) per month. Occasionally, allopathic medicines have been used in the Y group when deemed necessary, on a symptomatic basis.

The Y group received homoeopathic treatment, ranging from classical homoeopathy to combination therapies. The personalized prescriptions of the classical method took into account the present pathological state, as well as their mental, emotional, and physical characteristics, combined with familial histories and past clinical presentations. The classical prescriptions were made of the homoeopathic medicines whose pathogenesis was most similar to the totality of symptoms of the given individual. All of the medicines prescribed to the Y-group are recognized by the Food and Drug Administration of India under the Homoeopathic Pharmacopoeia. The diet of the Y group was similar to that of the X group as both were informed to eat protein rich foods that are easily digested, such as eggs, peas, and beans.

Data Collection

The management of the patient's condition was analyzed using a rapid evaluation technique, combining qualitative and quantitative data collection and analysis. The general condition and diagnosis were assessed by the attending physician, and thus, decision analysis was accepted. A retrospective record review was conducted at each site using a representative sample of patient records ($n=40$). The case records were randomly acquired to avoid bias. The health personnel at both sites were interviewed about the procedures and common practice management in relation to HIV+ patients, including aspects of HIV awareness and health promotion.

It is not possible to conduct a study such as this under cross-, double-, or blind methods, as that would entail denying medicines that empirically act favorably on the HIV individuals, from half of the test group. This would not be ethical as these patients are reaching out for any viable therapy. Therefore a retrospective analysis was used, as would be the case in an open- arms style study, now considered favorable in HIV studies.

Analysis of the Data:

The data was analyzed for several different criteria:

1) The initial assessment to determine that the patients were symptomatic at the beginning of treatment.
2) The progressive health or deterioration of the patient. The proportion of patients whose health was maintained being or well- controlled. For the purpose of this study, the physician's diagnosis as to whether the patient was deteriorating in health or benefiting from treatment was taken into consideration.

Table 2.1 : Health status at conclusion of study, including duration of treatment.

Patient No.	Age (At the time of diagnosis)	Date of diagnosis (month/year)	Date of death	Period between diagnosis & death	by attending physician
X1	32	2/99			Deteriorating
X2	30	3/99			Deteriorating
X3	35	8/99	09/99	1month	Expired
X4	40	5/98			Deteriorating
X5	45	12/98			Deteriorating
X6	25	1/98			Deteriorating
X7	42	6/98	09/99	15months	Expired
X8	32	6/98	12/98	6months	Expired
X9	35	10/98	11/98	1month	Expired
X10	22	8/97			Asymptomatic
X11	32	10/98	03/99	5months	Expired
X12	40	11/98	12/98	1month	Expired
X13	40	6/98			Asymptomatic
X14	34	10/98			Asymptomatic
X15	30	8/99			Deteriorating

Continue

Case Study

Patient No.	Age (At the time of diagnosis)	Date of diagnosis (month/year)	Date of death	Period between diagnosis&death	by attending physician
X16	20	2/99			Asymptomatic
X17	35	1/97	07/99	30months	Expired
X18	40	2/98	02/99	12months	Expired
X19	38	9/97	04/98	7months	Expired
X20	65	8/99	09/99	1month	Expired
Y1	27	12/96			Asymptomatic
Y2	47	5/95			Asymptomatic
Y3	35	6/95	08/99	50months	Expired
Y4	27	2/99			Asymptomatic
Y5	42	11/96			Asymptomatic
Y6	31	11/96			Asymptomatic
Y7	7	11/96			Asymptomatic
Y8	31	10/98			Asymptomatic
Y9	32	11/96			Asymptomatic
Y10	30	12/98			Asymptomatic
Y11	30	2/99			Asymptomatic
Y12	39	10/97	06/99	20months	Expired

Continue

Patient No.	Age (At the time of diagnosis)	Date of diagnosis (month/year)	Date of death	Period between diagnosis&death	by attending physician
Y13	24	5/99			Asymptomatic
Y14	8	4/98			Asymptomatic
Y15	27	5/99			Asymptomatic
Y16	32	3/98			Asymptomatic
Y17	39	4/99			Asymptomatic
Y18	47	12/98			Asymptomatic
Y19	35	1/99			Asymptomatic
Y20	37	11/97			Asymptomatic

Case Study

3) The conclusive assessment to determine the health status of the individual at the conclusion of the study.

Results

Eighty five percent of Y- group are diagnosed as being asymptomatic. A further five percent of Y- group is said to be healthy, yet suffers occasional diarrhoea. Ten percent of Y- group expired. X- group suffered a fifty percent mortality rate. A further thirty- five percent were diagnosed with a general condition that is deteriorating, by the attending physician. The remaining twenty percent were determined by the physician as being asymptomatic.

Table 2.2

Percentage Totals	X- group	Y- group
Expired	50%	10%
Deteriorating	30%	0%
Aysmptomatic	20%	90%

Table 2.3

Average length of time under treatment from date of diagnosis to date of death, if expired, or to present.

X- group	Y-group
9.5 months	21 months

Discussion and Observations:

Of the two patients who expired from Y- group, one patient lived a total of 50 months, that is the second longest of any of the patients from both groups; however, the patient (Y3) suffered from depression. The other patient who passed away from Y group lived a total of 20 months, however, suffered emotional ridicule and abuse in the workplace from colleagues who knew of his health status. It has been observed in several patients that those maintaining good spirits are thriving. This is perhaps exemplified in the case of X20, who died of no apparent cause within weeks of diagnosis; the patient willed himself to die. The patients in Y group received varying doses of medicine, ranging from daily to biweekly doses. The patients of Y group experienced similar symptoms to those of the X-group at an initial time of diagnosis, however, the majority have since put on weight and all other symptoms are negligible. Regular meetings between the patients of Y- group and their health practitioner are maintained.

Due to financial constraints, regular CD4+ counts were not obtainable in most cases. However, as is observable in the case of Y1, CD4+ counts raised from 310 to 531 in a matter of three months, with haemoglobin raising from 3.2 to 11.25 gm%. Similarly in the case of Y2, the patients CD4+ count raised from 62 to 281 from October 15/98 to December 15/98, a matter of two months. It s interesting to note the case of Y6 whom had a CD4 count of 62 in February '97, yet remains in total health to present. Similarly, in December '96, patient Y9 had a CD4+ count of 66, yet remains in health today.

The patients from X group received similar allopathic treatment to Y group, however, the majority are not thriving. The occurrence of greater health in Y- group may occur for several reasons:

Case Study

- homoeopathy may have played a major role in maintaining immunological balance.
- many patients maintained a healthy outlook on their lives.

Perhaps the most plausible explanation for the Y- group thriving in comparison to X group is that the homoeopathic treatment was individualized for each patient, along with their counselling and recommended lifestyle changes.

Conclusion:

Clinical assessment of the individuals from Y- group indicated that they were thriving in comparison to X group. This improvement may be due to the homoeopathic regimen applied to the group. Homoeopathy, in its application to this group may play a role in the treatment and control of HIV infection and in slowing down the progression to AIDS. This study is consistent with other studies of similar association and maintains a high level of applicability. Further studies assessing a greater number of patients with homoeopathy a sole treatment, as it relates to the prolongment of the asymptomatic individual, needs to be performed. Studies indicating precise haematological status is the next logical step to be built into the investigative protocol.

References:

1) Kalk, W.J., Beattie, A., Price, M., Broomberg, J. *The management of diabetes at primary level in South Africa: the results of a facility based assessment.* Journal of the Royal Society of Health, 1998, 118 (6);338-345

2) Rastogi, D.P., Singh, V.P., Singh, V., Dey, S.K., Rao, K. *Homeopathy in HIV infection: a trial report of double-blind placebo controlled study,* British Homoeopathic

Journal (1999)88, 49-57

3) Rastogi, D.P., Singh, V.P., Singh, V. Dey, S.K., *Evaluation of homoeopathic therapy in 129 asymptomatic HIV carriers*, British Homoeopathic Journal (1993) 82, 4-8

4) Shah, C., *Public Health and Preventive Medicine in Canada*, University of Toronto Press, 1999

5) Sterlick, J. *AIDS, the Homoeopathic Challenge*, Dove, 1996, London

II
Annexure

MATERIA MEDICA

"Consumption"

As the vast majority of developing nations HIV+ve patients eventually develop long periods in the symptomatic tubercular stage, it is necessary to highlight indications of common and uncommon remedies indicated in symptomatic situations. This is by no means meant to replace careful study of the case, repertory, nor materia medica, rather highlights relevant mental and physical characteristic symptoms of remedies that should be considered. This section is termed *"Consumption"* due to the consuming nature of the disease as well as the relationship to the Tubercular miasm.

Acalypha Indica

MIND, Despair, unwilling to die, in hemoptysis
MIND, Sadness, despondency, dejection, mental depression, gloom, melancholy

Marked action on the alimentary canal and respiratory organs. Incipient phthisis with hard, hacking cough, bloody expectoration, bright red hemoptysis. Blood bright red and not profuse in morning, rather dark and clotted in afternoon. Weak in morning, all symptoms worse in morning. Diarrhoea spluttering with forcible expulsion of noisy flatus. Jaundice. Furuncles.

Agaricin

Quotidian intermittent fevers, night sweats; hectic chills and fevers. Thick yellow coating of tongue. Aching of joints and small of back.

Agnus Cactus

    DREAMS - AMOROUS
    DREAMS - ANXIOUS
    DREAMS - FRIGHTFUL
    DREAMS - MANY
    MIND - DEATH - thoughts of
    MIND - DELIRIUM
    MIND - DELUSIONS - alarm, of - waking, on
    MIND - DELUSIONS - atmosphere - heavy and thick; atmosphere in room were
    MIND - DELUSIONS - awakened; he is - fright or alarm; awakened in
    MIND - DELUSIONS - dead - he himself was
    MIND - DELUSIONS - die - about to die; he was
    MIND - DELUSIONS - existence - doubt if anything had existence
    MIND - DELUSIONS - existence - surroundings did not exist
    MIND - DELUSIONS - head - fall; head would more - forward
    MIND - DELUSIONS - nobody; being
    MIND - DELUSIONS - smell, of
    MIND - DELUSIONS - turn - everything turned - circle;
    MIND - DELUSIONS - wealth, of

MIND - DEMENTIA - masturbation, with

This is a remedy which has marked action upon the sexuality of the individual, often to the point of perversions; later to result in a lapse of sexual energy and loss of body fluids. In the later stages, Agnus Castus presents a picture similar to AIDS. "Eventually these people begin to realize that their whole constitution is deteriorating. They feel a kind of dullness in the head. They feel old in their mind and body. In addition, they become impotent and suffer great preoccupation with this problem. They become convinced that they are about to have a nervous breakdown or that their vital organs are about to fail. This concern in Agnus castus becomes so great as to assume the proportions of significant anxiety about health. But these same people, as soon as they are alone, will think about their vices, the masturbation towards which they are extremely prone, and will become dissatisfied, discontented, and despise themselves."[1]

General weakness as a result of violent anguish, from depression.

Illusions of imaginary odors, as of herring, fishbrine, fermented beer or agreeable odors like musk.

Offensive flatus having ammonia-like odor or smelling like old urine.

Coldness of the genitalia with weakness, loss of sexual desire, loss of erections and decreased amount of semen. Testes cold, swollen, hard, and painful. Testes objectively cold at night.

Menses too late, scanty, absent or suppressed.

Perspiration during sleep.

Repeated attacks of gonorrhea.

Gouty joints. Rheumatic pains

Agraphis Nutans

Enlarged lymph nods. Catarrhal obstruction, adenoids. Tendency to take cold. Mucus diarrhoea worse in cold.

Allium Sativa

    MIND, Company, desire for, aversion to solitude
    MIND, Escape, desire to
    MIND, Fear, alone, being
    MIND, Fear, medicine, taking too much, fear of
    MIND, Fear, poisoned, he is
    MIND, Gluttony
    MIND, Impulse, morbid, run to, droromania
    MIND, Weeping, sleep, in
    DREAMS, Anxious (distressing, frightful, nightmares, sleep anxious, unpleasant)
    DREAMS, Storms
    DREAMS, Continuation of dreams after waking
    DREAMS, Journey, rapid transit, of
    DREAMS, Intellectual
    DREAMS, water, of

Frequent diarrhoea. Pulmonary TB patients who eat a lot. Rattling of mucus and rhonchi. Cough in the morning on leaving the room. Darting pains in chest. Expectoration dark and difficult. Weight loss. Irregular sleep. "Affects flesh eating animals and hardly ever vegetarians" (Teste).

Alumina

    MIND, Ailments from, sexual excesses
    MIND, Anxiety, conscience, as if guilty of a crime
    MIND, Blood, or a knife, cannot bear to look at

MIND, Censorious
MIND, Company, aversion to, presence of others
MIND, Confusion, identity, as to his
MIND, Courageous
MIND, Despair, recover, of
MIND, Dipsomania
MIND, Fear, disease, incurable, of being
MIND, Fear, evil, of evening
MIND, Fear, insanity, losing his reason
MIND, Fear, suicide, of
MIND, Fear, water, of
MIND, Kill, knife, at sight of, or a gun
MIND, Obscene, lewd
MIND, Shrieking, sleep, during
MIND, Suicidal, hypochondriasis by
MIND, Weeping, spasmodic
DELUSIONS, Crime, he had committed a
DELUSIONS, Dead persons, seeing
DELUSIONS, Fire, visions of
DELUSIONS, Specters, ghosts, spirits
DREAMS, Accidents, of, boat foundering
DREAMS, Amorous
DREAMS, Animals, horses, pursuing him
DREAMS, Animals, wild, pursued by
DREAMS, Snakes, Vermin, Worms
DREAMS, Cares, full of
DREAMS, Danger, falling
DREAMS, Dead, of the
DREAMS, Death
DREAMS, Dead, bodies
DREAMS, Drowning
DREAMS, Funerals
DREAMS, Humiliation

DREAMS, Meat, thrust into mouth
DREAMS, Sailing
DREAMS, Wading, water, in with snakes
DREAMS, Water (bathing, danger, drowning, falling, fishes, flood, sailing, sea, swimming, stream)

Dysphagia. Dryness and constriction throughout body. Haemorrhage of bowels. Weakness of muscles in all parts of body. Enlarged tonsils, burning pains in oesophagus. Haemoptysis with weakness of chest. Copious expectoration worse in morning. Induration and hardening of glands, with tendency to ulceration. Palpitation of heart, worse lying right sided. Ulcerations on skin, purple lesions, varicosities, alopecia.

Ammonium Causticum

MIND - ANGUISH
MIND - FRIGHTENED easily
MIND - IRRITABILITY
MIND - RESTLESSNESS - night
MIND - TIMIDITY
MIND - UNCONSCIOUSNESS
EYE - BLEEDING from eyes

Vithoulkas[2]: There is also marked exhaustion and muscular debility, indicating that this remedy should be considered for neuromuscular diseases, especially when one of the primary presenting symptoms is difficult deglutition (eating). These patients suffer oppression of the chest with anguish; they feel that they cannot take a breath, that they are suffocating. There is great difficulty in breathing."

This remedy is a powerful cardiac stimulant. As such, in syncope, thrombosis, haemorrhage, chloroform narcosis. The oedema and ulceration of mucous membranes produced by this powerful drug have been utilized as guiding symptoms for its use; hence its use in membranous croup with burning in the oesophagus. Aphonia.

Sleep results in a suffocating feeling. There is a strong tendency to affect the epithelium of the upper digestive tract. The tongue, the palate, and the esophagus are whitish and partially covered with blisters. White patches occur on the tongue and the inner side of the cheeks, reminding one of the symptoms of AIDS. Actually, the entire picture of this remedy in its extreme prostration, the emaciation, the effect upon the respiratory system and the mucous membranes, the arthritic pains, etc. suggests its probable usefulness for patients with AIDS. Hemorrhages particularly of the mucous membranes, with a tendency to faint.

Of note on the emotional level is a remarkable timidity with a tendency to be easily frightened. There may be great excitement in the evening. The face wears an expression of great anxiety, even anguish. There is also despair. (Vithoulkas)

White patches on the tongue and inner side of cheeks.

Vomiting of mucus and blood. Violent ejection of stomach contents from mouth and nose. Burning in oesophagus. Dark vomitus.

Voice lost, aphonia. Bronchitis with profuse expectoration, blood-stained. Respiration stridulous; rattling. Oppression with great difficulty in breathing; gasping for breath. Cough, ameliorated by cold drinks. Cough and much expectoration, especially after drinking. Sensation as if a foreign body were in the larynx. Mucus in larynx. Persistent cough. Spasmodic cough. Expectoration when liquids come into contact with posterior pharynx. Bloody expectoration.

Anantherum

MIND - AILMENTS FROM - anger
MIND - AILMENTS FROM - debauchery
MIND - AMOROUS
MIND - INSANITY, madness - masturbation, from
MIND - INSANITY, madness - sexual excesses, from
MIND - IRRITABILITY
MIND - JEALOUSY
MIND - LAUGHING
MIND - MANIA
MIND - STUPEFACTION
MIND - SUICIDAL disposition
MIND - SUSPICIOUS
MIND - SYMPATHETIC
MIND - TRAVELLING - desire for
MIND - WEEPING
DREAMS - DISEASE
DREAMS - DISEASE - hydrophobia
DREAMS - FALLING - height, from a
DREAMS - FEASTING
DREAMS - JOURNEYS
DREAMS - QUARRELS

This remedy has not been well known. Recently however, Vithoulkas described his observations of the remedy in his book <u>Materia Medica Viva</u>[3].

"Anantherum is a remedy that stimulates the lower passions of man, most specifically the sexual passions, to such excess that an individual so affected may be driven mad by the sheer force of his desire. This is a remedy that may be seen more and more these days. It creates an insatiable desire to satisfy the sexual urge, driving the person to repeated sexual contacts. If this urge cannot be satisfied, he is driven to masturbation. The desire is pathological, indicative of an organism completely out of check, impulsively driven to actions which could very well lead to its rapid self-destruction. It must be acknowledged that this remedy will find special application in that subset of homosexuals exhibiting such intensity of sexual behaviour. For these individuals sexual satisfaction lies above all other concerns. They seem to be exclusively driven by their unlimited sexual urges, perhaps having two or even three sexual liaisons during the day. Venereal appetite increased by every attempt to satisfy it until driven to onanism and madness. This remedy can induce the desire to dress publicly in a peculiar, grotesque manner, all the while hoping to impress others with their shocking appearance. It must be understood that the sexual excitement is tremendous, literally driving the helpless individual to pursue sexual contact. There is violent desire with violent erections, even priapism. It is a state of monomania.

Ulceration of margins of lids. In the face we see miliary eruptions, urticaria, pimples, eruptions which are crusty, scabby eruptions, herpetic eruptions; miliary and urticarious eruptions; erysipelatous swelling; abscess.

Tympanitic distension. Dropsy, edema. Inflammation and swelling of liver

Large hemorrhoidal tumors and abscesses

Sensation as if the urethral canal was obstructed by tumors and excrescences.

Syphilitic ulcers

Diseased and distorted nails

Dreams of epidemics, contagious diseases and especially of hydrophobia.

Arsenicum lodatum

MIND - DELUSIONS
MIND - DELUSIONS - dead - persons, sees
MIND - DELUSIONS - fancy, illusions of
MIND - DESPAIR
DREAMS, Amorous
DREAMS, Dead, of the
DREAMS, Frightful (anxious)
DREAMS, Nightmares (sleep anxious)
DREAMS, Vivid

It seems probable that in Ars. iod. we have a remedy most closely allied to manifestations of tuberculosis. It will be indicated by profound prostration, rapid, irritable pulse, recurring fever and night sweats, emaciation; tendency to diarrhoea. Chronic pneumonia, with abscess in lung. Hectic; debility; nightsweats(Boericke)[4].

It should be well noted that this is, perhaps along with Tuberculinum, the most indicated remedy in HIV.

Induration is a strong feature, in glands, in ulcers, in skin affections. Inflammation of glands, bones and serous membranes. Hodgkin's disease. Sarcoidosis. Affecting all glands, liver, spleen and thyroid gland. The face looks sickly, old, tired with bluish lips and bluish circles around eyes.

Baryta Carbonica

- MIND, Ailments from, anger
- MIND, Ailments from, anticipation
- MIND, Biting nails
- MIND, Childish behaviour, in old age
- MIND, Company, aversion to, presence of others
- MIND, Dementia senilis
- MIND, Fear, of death
- MIND, Frightened easily
- MIND, Imbecility
- MIND, Infantile behaviour
- MIND, Irresolution, indecision
- MIND, Malicious, spiteful
- MIND, Rage, trifles, at
- MIND, Sensitive, to sensual impressions
- MIND, Weeping, whimpering, sleep during
- DELUSIONS, Deserted, forsaken, he is
- DELUSIONS, Criticized, he is
- DELUSIONS, Fire, every noise is cry of fire
- DELUSIONS, people looking at him
- DREAMS, Amorous
- DREAMS, Dead, of the
- DREAMS, Dead bodies
- DREAMS, Disease
- DREAMS, Hideous
- DREAMS, Misfortune (accidents, disaster, events unfortunate, loss)
- DREAMS, Visionary

Scrofulous. Strong fear of strangers. Indurated glands: testes, occipital, submaxilliary, mesenteric. Quinsy. Dry suffocative cough. Chronic catarrhal states and T.B.. Chest is full of mucus but lacks strength to expectorate. Night sweats, twitching in sleep. Dyspepsia. Ailments from abuse of sex and fantasies.

Blatta Orientalis

Cough with dyspnoea in bronchitis, phthisis. Much pus like mucus. Indicated after Arsenicum.

Borax

    MIND, Abusive, insulting
    MIND, Anxiety, motion, downwards -motion, any.
    MIND, Clinging (to persons or furniture)
    MIND, Fear, falling
    MIND, Thunderstorms
    MIND, Laughing
    MIND, Rebels, against poultices
    MIND, Slander, disposition to
    MIND, Starting, easily
    MIND, Violent
    MIND, Weeping, sleep, in
    DELUSIONS, Possessed, devils, by
    DREAMS, Amorous (coition)
    DREAMS, Frightful
    DREAMS, Vexatious

Anxiety and fear being carried, especially down stairs. G.I. irritation, salivation, nausea, vomiting, colic, diarrhoea, collapse, spasms. Aphtous ulcerations, thrush, candidiasis: expectoration mouldy. Pleurodynia, worse upper right lobe. Herpes zoster, dermatomes. Night sweats, especially on head.

Boletus Laricus

MIND, Bilious disposition
MIND, Change, dislike of
MIND, Irritability
MIND, Restlessness, night
DREAMS, Frightful
DREAMS, Water

Intermittent fever. Night sweats. Hectic fever. Chilliness along spine with intense heat. Nausea. Pruritis.

Bromium

MIND - DELUSIONS - dead - persons, sees
MIND - DELUSIONS - images, phantoms; sees
MIND - DELUSIONS - insane - become insane; he will
MIND - DELUSIONS - looking - someone is looking - shoulder; over her
MIND - DELUSIONS - specters, ghosts, spirits - evening - appear; a specter will
MIND - DELUSIONS - strangers - looking over shoulder
MIND - HYSTERIA - sexual - excitement; from suppression of sexual
MIND - INDIFFERENCE, apathy - household affairs
DREAMS − COFFINS
DREAMS - DEATH - dying - he is
DREAMS - EXERTION; of physical
DREAMS - FIGHTS
DREAMS − FUNERALS

Tendency to infiltrate glands, become hard. Nose, tickling, smarting, as of cobwebs. Dry cough, with hoarseness and burning pains behind sternum. Spasmodic cough, with rattling of mucous in the larynx. Cold sensation when inspiring. Glands stony hard, especially on lower jaw and throat. Acne, pimples, boils, pustules. Worse from evening until midnight, and when sitting in a warm room; warm, damp weather, when at rest and lying on left side. Better, from any motion; exercise; at sea.

Calcarea Fluorica

MIND, Anxiety, money matters, about
MIND, Avarice
MIND, Fear, misfortune, of
MIND, Industrious, desire for work
MIND, Ideas, abundant, clearness of mind
DELUSIONS, Poor, he is
DELUSIONS, Want, he will come to
DREAMS, Cutting
DREAMS, Danger, impending
DREAMS, Dead, of the
DREAMS, Dead people, weeping with
DREAMS, Death
DREAMS, Death, relatives, of
DREAMS, Journeys (difficult, foreign country)
DREAMS, Weeping
DREAMS, Window, trying to get out of, from a dream

Nutritional deficiency. Depression. Hard, stony glands, infected and inflamed. Mouth and throat ulcerations, loose teeth. Cough with tiny lumps of yellow mucus with tickling cough and worse lying down. Bleeding from lungs. Endocardial fibroid deposits. Exhausting night sweats. Purple raised lesions. Malnutrition of bones. Cataracts, keratitis Subcutaneous cysts. Vomiting of undigested foods. Gout. History of syphilis.

Calcarea Phosphorica

MIND, Ailments from, anger, vexation
MIND, Ailments from, love, disappointed
MIND, Ailments from, sexual excesses
MIND, Cares, worries, full of
MIND, Clinging, wants to be held
MIND, Company, desire for, aversion to solitude
MIND, Contradiction, is intolerant of
MIND, Cretinism
MIND, Dementia senilis
MIND, Discontented, displeased, dissatisfied
MIND, Fear, disease, cancer, of
MIND, Fear, evil, of
MIND, Indignation
MIND, Industrious, mania for work
MIND, Lascivious (Lustful)
MIND, Nymphomania
MIND, Reproaches himself -Others
MIND, Sadness, anger, from
MIND, Wildness, unpleasant news, from
DELUSIONS, Fire, visions of
DELUSION, Home, away from, must get there
DREAMS, Amorous
DREAMS, Animals, of cats, army of
DREAMS, Difficulties, on journeys
DREAMS, Journeys (Difficulties, foreign countries)
DREAMS, Fire

Most often to be used when Phos. is indicated in T.B. patients to avoid serious aggravations. Anaemia with T.B., cough lying down, left lobe. Swollen glands, adenoids, lymph. Profuse perspiration. Diarrhoea worse from fruits; foetid.

Hoarseness of voice. Wasting, slimming disease. Worse from change of weather.

Calcarea Silicata

MIND, Ailments from, sexual excesses
MIND, Ambition, loss of
MIND, Anxiety, health about
MIND, Discontented. everything, with
MIND, Fear, brain, of softening of
MIND, Fear, disease, incurable, of being
MIND, Fear, of touch
MIND, Talks, dead people, with
MIND, Yielding, disposition
DELUSIONS, Dogs, sees
DELUSIONS, Dead persons, sees
DELUSIONS, People, disagreeable, sees
DELUSIONS, Faces, hideous
DELUSIONS, Starve, family will
DELUSIONS, Visions, has terrible
DREAMS, Amorous
DREAMS, Anxious
DREAMS, Dead, of the
DREAMS, Dead bodies
DREAMS, Death
DREAMS, Fire
DREAMS, Frightful
DREAMS, Murder (Killing)
DREAMS, Sick people
DREAMS, Vexatious
DREAMS, Visionary

Fearful. Complaints come on slowly and reach final development after a long time. Sensitive to cold. Chilly patient but worse on being overheated. Weak and emaciated. Pain in chest walls with copious yellow, green mucus.

Calotropis

MIND, Restlessness, night

Used in syphilis, elephantiasis, leprosy, acute dysentery. Pneumonic T.B.. T.B. of the syphilitic miasm if mercury cannot be used any further. Flesh decreases, muscles harden and firm. Heat in stomach. Anaemia.

Carbo Vegetabalis

MIND, Ailments from, sexual excesses
MIND, Ailments from, debauchery
MIND, Anguish
MIND, Answers, incorrectly
MIND, Anxiety, evening, bed, in
MIND, Anxiety, conscience (as if guilty of a crime)
MIND, Beside oneself, being
MIND, Clinging, restlessness, with
MIND, Confusion, as in a dream
MIND, Death, desires
MIND, Doubtful
MIND, Fear, evil, of
MIND, Fear, ghosts
MIND, Fear, happen, something will
MIND, Fear, overpowering
MIND, Kicks, worm affection, in
MIND, Liar
MIND, Libertinism

MIND, Music, palpitation on listening to
MIND, Nymphomania
MIND, Obscene, lewd
MIND, Offended easily, takes everything in bad part
MIND, Rage, in worm affections
MIND, Spying, everything
MIND, Suicidal, shooting, hanging
MIND, Weeping, sad thought, at
DELUSIONS, Anxious
DELUSIONS, Crime, he had committed a
DELUSIONS, Deserted, forsaken, is
DELUSIONS, Hand, passes over body
DELUSIONS, Visions, horrible, has
DREAMS, Amorous
DREAMS, Fire
DREAMS, Ghosts, specters
DREAMS, Lewd, lascivious, voluptuous
DREAMS, Music
DREAMS, Scientific
DREAMS, Water

Disintegration and imperfect oxidation. Lowered vital power from overdrugging. Burning in the chest with haemoptysis. Spasmodic cough with gagging and vomiting of mucus. Lifeless body with a hot head. Hoarseness especially in the evening. Haemorrhage from lungs, and mucus membranes. Debilitated. Hectic fever with exhausting sweats. Coldness, blueness. Better in air, cold. Never better since previous illness. Flatulence. Bleeding rectum, cadaverous stools.

China Arsenicum

MIND, Ailments from, sexual excesses
MIND, Censorious

MIND, Confusion (of mind)
MIND, Fear, disease, cancer, of
MIND, Fear, ghosts, at night
MIND, Loathing of life
MIND, Sensitive (oversensitive)
MIND, Talk, indisposed to, desire to be silent, taciturn
DELUSIONS, Fancy, of
DELUSIONS, Images, frightful
DELUSIONS, Prostration, cannot endure such
DREAMS, Death
DREAMS, Emotional causes, from
DREAMS, Misfortune (accidents, disaster, events, unfortunate, loss)

Weariness and sudden prostration. Dyspnoea with profuse sweat. Eggs produce diarrhoea. Icy skin.

Eriodictyon

MIND, Exhilaration
MIND, Memory, weakness of
MIND, Moaning, sleep, during
DREAMS, Anxious

Appetite poor. Impaired digestion. Foul breath especially in the morning. Chronic bronchitis and bronchial T.B. with profuse easily raised bronchial secretions. Dull pain in right lung. Night sweats and emaciation.

Ferrum Arsenicum

MIND, Anxiety, conscience (as if guilty of a crime)
MIND, Death, thoughts of

MIND, Fear, death
    -evil
    -people
    -misfortune
MIND, Obstinate (headstrong)
MIND, Religious affections
MIND, Tranquility (serenity, calmness)
DREAMS, Anxious

Phthisis with enlarged spleen and liver. Pernicious anemia. Chlorosis. Enlarged spleen and liver. Undigested stool. Albuminuria.

Ferrum Phosphoricum

MIND, Ailments from, anger, vexation
MIND, Company, aversion, alone, >alone
MIND, Courageous
MIND, Fear, apoplexy
MIND, Fear, crowd, in a
MIND, Fear, Death
MIND, Fear, evil, of
MIND, Hypochondriasis
MIND, Hysteria
MIND, Loquacity
MIND, Restlessness, bed, driving out of
MIND, Shrieking
MIND, Singing
DREAMS, Confused (disconnected)
DREAMS, Disease, insane, becoming
DREAMS, Falling
DREAMS, Insane, becoming
DREAMS, Nightmares

DREAMS, Quarrels (abused, anger, insults, provoked, reconciliation)

Often to be used when Phos. is indicated. Nervous, sensitive anemic type, with false plethora. Palliates acute exacerbation of T.B. Epistaxis. Facial neuralgia. Hematemesis. Congestion of lungs, hemoptysis, expectoration of pure blood (bright red), better at night. Hard, dry cough with sore chest. Meningitis, stiff neck. Night sweats. Chill at 1pm. Pulse soft.

Formic Acid

Gouty diathesis (myositis, periostitic processes, fascitis). History of STD's. Encephalitis. Failing vision. Fatigue and tremor. T.B. with nephritis, arthritis. Immunity disordered, carcinomas.

Formica Rufa

MIND, Activity, mental
MIND, Ailments from, mortification
MIND, Eccentricity
MIND, Bad news, after
MIND, Morose (cross, peevish, ill humor, fretful)
DREAMS, Amorous
DREAMS, Coffins (funerals)
DREAMS, Funerals (churchyard, coffins, graves)
DREAMS, Lewd, lascivious

Gouty diathesis. Tendency to take cold, worse at night. Pleuritic pains. T.B., cancers, autoimmune disorders. Gas is trapped. Hoarseness with dry sore throat. Vomiting yellow mucus.

Fluoric Acid

MIND, Ailments from, debauchery
MIND, Ailments from, mental work
MIND, Aversion, members of his family
MIND, Business, aversion to
MIND, Deceitful (sly)
MIND, Ecstasy
MIND, Fancies, exhaltation of
MIND, Fear, death, of
MIND, Forgetful, wind his watch, to
MIND, Industrious (mania for work)
MIND, Insanity, immobile as a statue
MIND, Mannish habits, of women
MIND, Mistakes, localities in
MIND, Rage (fury)
MIND, Nymphomania
MIND, Thoughts, rush, flow out
MIND, Walking rapidly, from anxiety
DELUSIONS, Betrothal must be broken
DELUSIONS, Dead persons, sees
DELUSIONS, Images, when alone
DELUSIONS, Repulsive, fantastic
DELUSIONS, Danger, impression of
DREAMS, Acquaintances, distant
DREAMS, Dead relatives
DREAMS, Death- himself, orders the rapid removal of the corpse from the house
DREAMS, Death- of a friend
DREAMS, Death, relatives, of
DREAMS, Fire
DREAMS, Frightful
DREAMS, Remorses (religious, reproaches)

History of syphilis. Indifference to loved ones. Mood swings. Deep destruction of tissues. Bedsores, ulcerations, distended blood vessels, Kaposi's sarcoma. Hob nailed liver. Nightly fevers. Dyspnoea. Hydrothorax.

Guaiacol

DREAMS, Battles
DREAMS, Cut (being)
DREAMS, Falling, height, from a
DREAMS, Hideous
DREAMS, Misfortune (accidents, disaster, events unfortunate, loss)
DREAMS, Murdered, being
DREAMS, Nightmares
DREAMS, Riots (insurrections, revolution)
DREAMS, Scientific
DREAMS, Stabbed, being

Secondary syphilis, gout. Odour from the whole body. Contraction of limbs. Pleuritic pains, suffocative. Constriction of epigastrium. Stiff neck and shoulders.

Hippozaenium (Nosode of glanders)

MIND, Delirium

AIDS, syphilis, cancer, T.B.. Ozaena, scrofulous swellings, pyemia, erysipelas, saneous secretion. Tubercles throughout the body. T.B. with chronic cavity in lung. Excessive expectoration producing noisy breathing. Ulceration of frontal sinus and pharynx. Inflamed glands, lymphs. Nodules in arm. Articular, non- fluctuating swellings. This nosode covers symptoms which suggest its integral use in end stage AIDS.

Iodum

MIND - AILMENTS FROM - fright
MIND - AILMENTS FROM - love; disappointed
MIND - AILMENTS FROM - mental exertion
MIND - AILMENTS FROM - mental shock; from
MIND - AILMENTS FROM - sexual - excesses
MIND - AMOROUS
MIND - DELUSIONS - dead - persons, sees
MIND - DELUSIONS - falling - walking; when - if she walks
MIND - DELUSIONS - fancy, illusions of
MIND - DELUSIONS - insane - become insane; he will
MIND - DELUSIONS - iodine; illusions of fumes of
MIND - DELUSIONS - sick - being
MIND - DELUSIONS - water - of
MIND - DELUSIONS - well, he is
MIND - DELUSIONS- fasting
MIND, DELUSIONS- insane, become, that she will
MIND - DELUSIONS- sick, he is
MIND, DELUSIONS- well, he is
MIND - DESPAIR
MIND - DESTRUCTIVENESS
MIND - FEAR - death, of
MIND - FEAR - doctors
MIND - FEAR - evil; fear of
MIND - FEAR - failure, of
MIND - KILL; desire to - woman; irresistible impulse to kill a
MIND- Destructiveness
MIND- Fear, physician, will not see the, he seems to terrify her
MIND- Fear, disease, of impending
DREAMS; eating, excrements, wading in excrements

Materia Medica 169

DREAMS, Accidents (disaster, misfortune)
DREAMS, Amorous, pollutions, with
DREAMS, Dead, of the
DREAMS, Dead bodies
DREAMS, Disgusting, soiling himself with excrements
DREAMS, Eating
DREAMS, Excrements
DREAMS, Falling water into
DREAMS, Falling- water, into, daughter is
DREAMS, Misfortune
DREAMS, Swimming
DREAMS, Water

It is the knowledge of this remedy and its related drugs which will bring the greatest relief to the symptomatic patient. The understanding of this drug allows us to recognize the compatability towards the general picture of the middle stage HIV.

The patient is hurried in all actions, rapid and fast. This has a correlation with the thyroid and metabolism. Combustion, said by Vithoulkas to represent the essence of the remedy, can easily be understood as their actions require and use so much energy. Heat, the hottest of remedies, often with very hot night sweats. There is a loss of control with the restlessness and decisions are made so quickly that they are not thought out. The impulsiveness barely allows the patient to remain in the chair, the speech is quick and loquacious. There is sudden impulse, to kill, themselves or others. Compulsive neurosis about their health is observed and the patient may continually look for assurance. These compulsive behaviours result in exhaustion. Emaciation, as in the disease, is seen in this remedy with enlarged and hardened glands, enlarged liver, and spleen.

Candidiasis is observed along with haematological disorders. This remedy requires careful study as it presents a picture of AIDS.

Iodoform

    MIND, Cheerful (gay, mirthful)
    MIND, Delirium (in general)
    MIND, Eccentricity
    MIND, Loquacity
    MIND, Mania
    MIND, Shrieking (screaming, shouting)
    MIND, Suicidal disposition
    MIND, Violent, deeds of rage, leading to
    DREAMS, Accidents (disaster, misfortune)
    DREAMS, Confused (disconnected)

Sleep Interrupted by sighing and cries. Tuberculous condition especially used in tubercular meningitis. Cough and wheezing on going to bed, with hemoptysis. Chronic diarrhoea. Pain in apex of right lobe.

Kali Iodatum

    MIND, Ailments from, mental work
    MIND, Anger, violent
    MIND, Complaining
    MIND, Cruelty, inhumanity
    MIND, Disgust
    MIND, Fear, dawn, of the return
    MIND, Frightened easily
    MIND, Impetuous
    MIND, Malicious (in sadness)

Materia Medica 171

MIND, Passionate
MIND, Weeping, anxiety, after
MIND, Weeping, anxious
DREAMS, Danger
DREAMS, Falling
DREAMS, Frightful
DREAMS, Joyous
DREAMS, Murder (killing)
DREAMS, Murdered, being
DREAMS, Nightmares
MIND, DELUSIONS, specters, ghosts, spirits, sees
MIND, DELUSIONS, poisoned has been, he
MIND, DEMENTIA, syphilitics, of
MIND, FEAR, evil, of
MIND, Passionate
MIND, Sadness, fear, with, evil, of impending
MIND, Weeping, tearful mood, evil impended, as if

History of syphilis. In acute stage with evening remitting fever, going off in nightly perspiration. Second stage, mucus membranes and skin ulcerations. Third stage, tertiary symptoms, nodes. Thrush, ringworm. Syphilis and TB. Loss of weight and hemoptysis. Burning pains. Expectoration like soap suds, greenish. Stitching pains through lungs to back. Purple spots on skin. Glands enlarged, indurated. Fissured anus.

Manganum

MIND, Answers, aversion to
MIND, Confusion (of mind)
MIND, Embittered
MIND, Grief, future, for the
MIND, Hatred

MIND, Hysteria
MIND, Imbecility
MIND, Meditation
MIND, Music, aversion to joyous, immediately affected
MIND, Morose
MIND, Wearisome
DELUSIONS, Enlarged, head is
DELUSIONS, Images, frightful
DELUSION, Enlarged, body parts, are
DREAMS, Danger, death of
DREAMS, Events, future, prophetic
DREAMS, Frightful
DREAMS, Hideous
DREAMS, Joyous
DREAMS, Nightmares (sleep anxious)
DREAMS, Physician (disease, sick people)
DREAMS, Prophetic
DREAMS, Shot, being
DREAMS, Soldier
DREAMS, Vexatious

Anemia with destruction of the red corpuscles. Fatty degeneration of the liver. Early T.B. of larynx, chronic hoarseness. Cough worse in evening. Better lying down. Much accumulated mucus. Every cold has bronchitis. Feeble staggering gait. Gout. Red elevated spots on skin. Jaundice. Mouth ulcers. History of syphilis.

Kali Nitricum

MIND, Cares (worries full of)
MIND, Beside oneself, being
MIND, Death, presentiment of
MIND, Fear, death, of

MIND, Indifference, with apathy
MIND, Love, perversity
MIND, Offended easily, takes everything in bad part
Delusion: fingers are long
Delusion: fires
Delusion: penis breaks off
Delusion: face falls off
Delusion: is a leper
DREAMS, Amorous
DREAMS, Anger
DREAMS, Body emaciated, becoming
DREAMS, Body parts of, parts swollen
DREAMS, Body parts, penis breaking off
DREAMS, Body parts, teeth breaking off
DREAMS, Children being beaten
DREAMS, Danger, water from (flood)
DREAMS, Dead, of the
DREAMS, Death
DREAMS, Disease (Physician, sick people)
DREAMS, Disease, poisoning
DREAMS, Disease, swelling face
DREAMS, Disgusting
DREAMS, Falling
DREAMS, Fire
DREAMS, Journeys
DREAMS, Men, following to violate her
DREAMS, Nightmares
DREAMS, Poisoned, of being
DREAMS, Riots
DREAMS, Water

Sudden dropsical swellings of body. Inflammation with much debility, esp. in T.B. Expectorates clotted blood after hawking. Dyspnoea so great cannot drink. Nephritis. Ennui.

Lachnanthes

    MIND, Delirium, loquacious
    MIND, Cheerful
    DELUSIONS, Images, phantoms, specters
    DELUSIONS, Snakes in and around her
    MIND, Loquacity, stupid and irritable, then
    MIND, Moaning (groaning, whining)
    MIND, Touched, aversion to being
    DREAMS, Anxious
    DREAMS, Feverish
    DREAMS, Spinning
    DREAMS, Visionary

Light complexion. Desires to talk, make a speech. Early stages of T.B. and established chest cases. Loquacity. Circumscribed red cheeks. Tendency to sweat. Septic throats. Icy cold body, yet sweats.

Lactic Acid

    MIND, Censorious (critical)
    MIND, Contemptuous
    MIND, Eccentricity
    MIND, Fastidious
    MIND, Mocking, sarcasm
    MIND, Reading, aversion
    MIND, Sensitive, noise
    MIND, Thoughts, tormenting
    DREAMS, Amorous
    DREAMS, Coition, of, erections, with, but no erections
    DREAMS, Precipices (falling)
    DREAMS Precipices, abyss, in cramp

Tubercular ulceration of vocal cords as a lump or a puff ball in the throat, keeps swallowing. Pain in chest with enlarged axilliary glands, pain extends to hands.

Myrtus Communis

MIND, Discouraged

Incipient phthisis. Dry, hollow cough, tickling. Worse mornings. Sensation of burning in chest.

Naphthaline

History of gonorrhoea. Pulmonary T.B. Terribly offensive ammonical urine. Tenacious expectoration. Hay fever. Pyelonephritis. Worms, pin worms.

Nitric Acid

MIND, Abrupt, rough
MIND, Ailments from, grief
MIND, Abusive, insulting
MIND, Ailments from, discords with parents, family
- chief and subordinates
MIND, Ailments from, sexual excesses
MIND, Amorous
MIND, Anger, violent
MIND, Anxiety of conscience (as if guilty of a crime)
MIND, Delirium, raging, raving
MIND, Dementia of syphilitics
MIND, Despair
MIND, Discouraged, cursing with
MIND, Doubtful, recovery, of

MIND, Estranged, family, from her
MIND, Fear, cholera, of
MIND, Fear, death, of
MIND, Fear, disease, cancer, of
MIND, Fear, starting, with
MIND, Fear, weary of life, with
MIND, Homesickness
MIND, Ideas, deficiency of
MIND, Lascivious (lustful)
MIND, Malicious (spiteful, vindictive)
MIND, Moral feeling, want of
MIND, Philosophy, ability for
MIND, Rage (fury)
MIND, Resignation
MIND, Sadness
MIND, Sensitive, noise, stepping of
MIND, Shrieking, sleep, during
MIND, Spoken, aversion to being
DELUSIONS, Disease, incurable, has
DELUSIONS, Dead persons, sees
DELUSIONS, Die, he was about to
DELUSIONS, Images, frightful
DELUSIONS, Images, phantoms
DELUSIONS, Offended people, he has
DELUSIONS, Strangers, sees
DELUSIONS, Talking irrationally
DELUSIONS, Talking, insane
DREAMS, Accidents
DREAMS, Amorous
DREAMS, Banquet
DREAMS, Carousing
DREAMS, Continuation of dreams, after waking
DREAMS, Crime (guilt)

DREAMS, Dead, of the
DREAMS, Dead bodies
DREAMS, Frightful
DREAMS, Feasting (banquets)
DREAMS, Ghosts, specters
DREAMS, Lewd, lascivious
DREAMS, Nightmares
DREAMS, Sad (cares, weeping)
DREAMS, Visionary (fantastic)

History of syphilis, gonorrhoea. Fear of death, hopeless despair. Vindictive, hateful. Pain as of splinters, especially in mucus membranes. Blisters, ulcers in mouth, genitals- bleeding. Hoarseness, aphonia, with dry hacking cough, from tickling in larynx and pit of stomach, soreness at lower end of stomach. All discharges offensive, disposed to diarrhoea. Genital warts. For chronic ailments with cachexia, intermittent fevers, and liver involvement with anemia.

Phellandrium

MIND, Anxiety, health, about
MIND, Exhilaration
MIND, Extravagance
MIND, Hydrophobia
MIND, Loathing (general)
MIND, Weeping, sad thoughts, at
DREAMS, Fights (battles, duels, enemies, quarrels, stabbed, war, wounded)
DREAMS, Lightning
DREAMS, Sound in the brain, as if beating on a metal that was swinging freely, ameliorated 5 a.m.
DREAMS, Thunderstorms

Middle lobe T.B. with hemoptysis. Hectic diarrhoea. Cough compels to sit up. Desire for acids.

Pilocarpus Microphyllus

Night sweats. Profuse perspiration. Perspiration with salivation like white of an egg. Painless diarrhoea. Oedema of lungs. Enormous expectoration and perspiration.

Increased heart action and pulsation of arteries, tremors and nervousness. Nausea on looking at moving objects. Chilliness with sweats.

Spongia

    MIND, Anguish, Cardiac
    MIND, Anxiety, Dreams, on waking from frightful
    MIND, Anxiety, future, about
    MIND, Delirium, delusions, with
    MIND, Discontented, displeased, dissatisfied
    MIND, Disgust, everything, with
    MIND, Dwells, on past disagreeable circumstances
    MIND, Fear, death, of
    MIND, Fear, ghosts, of
    MIND. Fear, heart, disease of
    MIND, Fear, insanity, losing his reason
    MIND, Hypochondriasis
    MIND, Prostration (of mind, mental exhaustion, brain)
    MIND, Sadness, anxious
    MIND, Starting, sleep, from
    MIND, Weeping, heat, during
    DELUSIONS, Fancy (illusions of)
    DELUSIONS, Fire, visions of

DELUSIONS, Persecuted, he is
DELUSIONS, Pursued, tormented by frightful
DELUSIONS, Specters, closing eyes, on
DELUSIONS, Visions, has horrible, events, of past
DREAMS, Cares, full of
DREAMS, Dead, of the
DREAMS, Death
DREAMS, Fire
DREAMS, Frightful
DREAMS, Murder (killing)
DREAMS, Misfortune
DREAMS, Sad
DREAMS, Shooting
DREAMS, Visionary

Swollen glands. Anxiety and difficult breathing. The dry cough of heart involvement. Excitement increases cough. Cough dry, barking, larynx sensitive to touch. Hypertrophy of heart; heart feeble. Cough abates after eating or drinking.

Stannum Mettalicum

MIND, Ailments from, fright
MIND, Anger, talk, indisposed to
MIND, Answers, aversion to
MIND, Anxiety, future, about
MIND, Aversion, certain persons, to
MIND, Conversation <
MIND, Doubtful, recovery, of
MIND, Ecstasy
MIND, Exuberance
MIND, Fear, crowd, in a
MIND, Dear, death, of
MIND, Fear, jumps out of bed

MIND, Fear, people, of
MIND, Inconsolable
MIND, Irresolution, indecision
MIND, Industrious, mania for work
MIND, Laughing <
MIND, Mischievious
MIND, Reserved
MIND, Rest, desire to
MIND, Sadness (despondency, dejection, depression)
MIND, Speech, nonsensical
MIND, Weeping, involuntary
MIND, Weeping, nervous, feels like crying all the time
MIND, Talking, sleep, in
DELUSIONS, Disease, incurable, has
DELUSIONS, Lengthened, distances are
DELUSIONS, Fire, visions of
DREAMS, Accidents (explosions)
DREAMS, Amorous
DREAMS, Battles
DREAMS, Cruelty (ill treatment, mutilation, violence)
DREAMS, Fire
DREAMS, Fights, (battles, duels, enemies, quarrels, stabbed, war, wounded)
DREAMS, Hideous
DREAMS, Great
DREAMS, Misfortune
DREAMS, Monomania
DREAMS, Pleasant (joyous, peaceful, quiet, wonderful)
DREAMS, Riots
DREAMS, Splendour
DREAMS, Striving
DREAMS, Vivid
DREAMS, War (battles, air attacks, commanding, fights)

Debility. Dreads to see people, sadness, discouraged. T.B.. Hectic fever. Copious green, sweet expectoration. Cough excited by talking and laughing. Exhausting night sweats especially towards morning. Mucopurulent discharges. Adhesive mucus of throat. Bone pains. Pains come and go gradually. Limbs suddenly give out when attempting to sit down. Smell of cooking causes vomiting.

Syphilinum (Lueticum)

    MIND – ABUSIVE
    MIND – ANTISOCIAL
    MIND - DELUSIONS - dirty - he is
    MIND - DELUSIONS - insane - become insane; he will
    MIND - DELUSIONS - paralyzed; he is
    MIND - DESPAIR - recovery, of
    MIND – DISGUST
    MIND - FEAR - disease, of impending - incurable, of being
    MIND - FEAR - syphilis, of
    MIND - FEIGNING - sick; to be
    MIND - INDIFFERENCE, apathy - everything, to
    MIND - INDIFFERENCE, apathy - future, to
    MIND - INDIFFERENCE, apathy - loved ones, to
    MIND - INDIFFERENCE, apathy - pleasure, to
    MIND – SECRETIVE
    DREAMS - DISEASE - own disease, his

Utter prostration and debility in the morning. Alcoholism. Ulceration of mouth, nose, genitals, skin. Succession of abscesses. *Feels as if going insane or being paralyzed. Fears the night.* Tubercular iritis. Feeling of cold air blowing on the eye. Craves alcohol. Rheumatism of shoulder joint at the insertion of deltoid. Chronic asthma in summer. Lancinating pains from the base of the heart to the apex at night. Always washing the hands.

Tuberculin Miasm The Tuberculins:
Various Preparations:

Tuberculinum (Swan and Fincke)
Bacillinum (Burnett)
Tuberculinum (Koch's)
Tuberculinum (Koch's Residual)
Koch's Lymph
Aviare - *related as Mycobacterium Aviare Intracellulare is a common form of TB in AIDS*
Serum of Jousset
Allergen of Jousset
Dilute serum of Marmoreck
Tuberculinum Bovinum (Kent)
Human Tuberculin of Klebs.
Immunising bodies of Spengler
Dialysed Tuberculin
Autogenous products
Vaccine of Bossan
Serum of Movigliano
Pulverised Bacillary emulsion of Hallock
Vaccine of Vaudremer
Chloroformed Tuberculin
Bacilli of Osterman
Electronic Bacillinum of Whiting
Tuberculinum Porcinus
Bacillinum Testicum
Diluted B.C.G.
Serum of Ferran

Tuberculinum is the most indicated remedy in Indian HIV treatment. It is also the most indicated intercurrent remedy.

References:

Boericke, W., *Pocket Manual of Homoeopathic Materia Medica and Repertory*, B. Jain, Delhi, 1995

Dave, P.C. Homoeopath, Personal Interview, Oct 10th, 1999, Anand, Gujarat, India

Kent, J.T., *Lectures on Materia Medica*, B. Jain, Delhi, 1995

Master, F., *Homoeopathic Dictionary of Dreams*, B. Jain, Delhi, 1999

Master, F. *The Tuberculinum Miasm Tuberculins*, B. Jain, Delhi, 1997

Scholtan, J. *Elements and Homoeopathy*, Hompath Software, Mumbai, 1999

Tyler, M.L., *Homoeopathic Drug Pictures*, B. Jain, Delhi, 1995

Vithoulkas, G. *Materia Medica Viva*, Health and Habitat, Mill Valley, 1992

■■

III
Annexure

THEMES

Materia Medica Themes

Some years ago a trend came in homoeopathy to develop themes relating to remedies and the stages in disease. As has been previously examined the stages of disease are easily discernable. However, the stages of relative remedies is not as easily observed and much experience and communication between practitioners will be necessary before a reliable approach can be determined. However, certain themes are somewhat present and an attempt to explain them here will no doubt spur us towards better understanding and, at the very least, discussion.

The discussion that we will now attempt is by no means conclusive and should be wholly disregarded when actually working on a case. These examples are meant to merely begin thinking about the nature of this disease. Much of the ideas come from Dr. J. Scholten in his book *Homoeopathy and the Elements*. A further investigation of the associated thematic remedies will present an interesting progression.

Scholtan has dealt primarily with the elements of the periodic table and has linked them to certain stages of disease or health.

And as a result of this work he has presented a progression of remedies whose themes will often represent the stages of risk behaviour to eventual sickness. For the purpose of this paper, our attention can be directed towards the second column from the right down, from Fluorine (F), through Chlorum (Cl), to Bromum (Br), to Iodum (I), and finally with Astatinum (At). Examination of each remedy group will perhaps best exemplify these observations.

Fluorine Group (F)

The thematic picture of remedies in the Fluorine group represent perhaps the initial stages of risk behaviour. That is, risky behaviours and much breaking of moral opinions. The breaking of moral taboos and strict behaviours imposed on them results in behaviours such as sexuality or drug related. This can be beneficial in many ways to an individual in a stifling situation, however, for the purpose of this study, we will link it to high risk behaviours. However, this irate thinking may not be always discernable on the exterior and the habits may be done in secret, consider the visiting of a CSW. This group has a drive for the best of things, whether that be social scene, women, or material possessions. Taboo sexual issues such as homosexuality, sado masochism, CSW's, etc. are often a manner with which this group obtains their desires. This group paints an often seen picture of the modern jet set type. A strong desire to experience all things, yet related to a low self esteem which makes them attempt to live on the edge and for themselves. In the end we see a depressed state, worn out, and often infected.

Letting go of morals
Breaking Taboos

Glamour
Holding on to possessions
Quickly bored with their situation - desires change
Sexuality- perversions
Everything occurs fast, hurried
Narcissism
Letting go of their values
Lose the reason for living
Flee from themselves
Letting go of the ego
Banned because of egotism, sex, or who they are

Fears : life, strangers, future, travelling, flying, streets, failure, disease, operations, cancer, death, poverty, murder

Right sided
Warm

Desires : alcohol, spices, sour, refreshing
> Motion, violent motion
Lymph affections
Teeth caries and pains
Laryngitis, bronchitis, diptheria
Urethritis

Chlorum (Cl)

This remedy group have much in common with the patients that demand attention or sympathy. These patients are hypersensitive and demand so much attention that they cannot be pleased. There is much emotional sensitivity, seen also in their vivid dreams and hallucinations. The fears in this remedy reveal how the patient focuses on themselves and their sickness. The patients are apprehensive and irritable. There are many similarities in these remedies for the patients with a history of alcohol and drug abuse, as well as those using alcohol and drugs as a way to escape their situation. Another stage of this remedy presents prostration.

Banned because of their relationships and family
Everything or nothing
Loose
No integration
Me

Fears : night terrors, disease, insanity, poverty, water
Delirium tremens, mania a potu
Irritability, drinking wine and coffee, while
Stupefaction, as if intoxicated
Nymphomania
Fear, of impending disease
Fear, insanity, of losing his reason
Fear, poverty
Escape, attempts to
Delusion, insane become, that she will
Delusion, poisoned, has been, he
Delusion, want, will come to
Mania, madness, boisterous

Temperature moderate

Aphthae
Hemoptysis

Pleurisy
Tuberculosis
Ulcers

Bromum (Br)

The mental picture presented by this remedy can easily be related to many cases of middle to late stage HIV. The picture is as if they have been caught doing something wrong, as is often the case in HIV, they have been caught having done things not accepted by their society. This guilt is felt in many ways and the patient has so many wishes to regain his previous situation, before the problems began. There is a guiltiness in front of gods, as if they will be punished by god or this is a punishment. Work is a big issue with this group as they wish to get back to their progressive work periods where they are occupied and don't think of their present situation. This is exemplified by the rubric CHEST, ASTHMA, of sailors, when come ashore; that is, the patient has come back to their problems.

Work has come to an end
Letting go of work
Condemned, forced labour
Letting go of duty
Letting go of control: sex/ adultery
Feeling condemned and persecuted
Escaping after failure

Fears : failure, criticism, opposition, anticipation, alone, stroke, dark, ghosts, water

Dreams : unsuccessful efforts, paralysis, dead people,

funeral, travel, anger

> **Delusions :** someone looking over their shoulder
> **Delusions,** pursued
> **Delusions,** fasting
> **Delusions,** going insane
> **Delusions,** travelling
> **Delusions,** ghosts

Left

Warm
Swollen hard glandular affections
Thyroid affections
Cancerous affections
Skin diseases

Iodum (I)

These remedies are very much indicated in the late stage HIV patient. The restlessness and progressive pathology wear them out and they are left pondering their future. The themes of this remedy are indicative of their struggle to come to terms with the end of life. The idea that they are punished comes through and they are beginning to accept that they are not accepted. We see the rubric MIND, Ailments from, looked at, being. The struggle is observed in the delusions that he is sick or insane, or that he is well. MIND, Anxiety, when quiet, reveals how the patient concentrates on his situation, perceiving the end. The Iodum remedies have particular relevance in the treatment of the Tubercular state. Careful study of these remedies will provide much depth into the HIV patient. Iodum was used in its crude form in Eastern Europe immediately following the Chernobyl disaster to prevent complications of exposure to radiation. The pictures exist together, break down of immunity.

Loss of ambitions
Thoughts and memories jumbled
Obsessive
Sense of humor
Nothing matters anymore
Condemned because of ideas
Banned from their regions
Right of existence
Escape
Desires security

Fears : narrow spaces, failure, show, disasters, evil, hunger, trifles, disease, doctors, insanity, touch, looked at, held tight, water

Dreams : failure, prison, fleeing, fire, eating, walking in mud, water, accidents, erotic, feces, failed coition, ruins.

Right
Warm
Discharges acrid
Glands swollen and enlarged
Thyroid problems
Vocal affinities
Lung affections
Testes, ovaries, genitalia

Astatinum (At)

Astatinum has yet to be proven. Scholtan has postulated that the effects of Astatinum would be similar to the picture of final stage AIDS.

IV Annexure

CASE EXAMPLES

N.B. The following case examples of the homoeopathic treatment of HIV+ individuals were conducted by Dr. Farokh J. Master M.D. (Hom.). These case examples most readily highlight the necessity for constitutional treatment and proper case taking, giving importance to mental, emotional, physical, and pathological symptoms.

Case (I)

Patient J.B.F.
Initial consultation on 18-6-98
Age: 32
Male
Complaint: Nephrotic syndrome
Occupation: Lecturer
Family: Married with one son
Family history: Hypertension, TB, Cerebrovascular Accident
- Tubercular miasm

Symptoms

Nephrotic syndrome
- oedema over legs < evening
- oedema over face < morning

Sensitive to the smell of alcohol
- causes nausea and headache

Erythematous patches- started on ankles
- reached buttocks, then forearm
- pus formation
- leaves black scars

Desires red onions, raw, warm food

Aversion to fish

Headaches in sun
- from loss of sleep

Was "framed" by a professor at his college- humiliation++

Felt neglected at school ++

Conscientious about physical appearance +++
- "I have to be presentable"
- fond of clothes
- wants to be appreciated +++

Fear of bad news relating to his son

Jealous of people who look better than him+++

Wanted to be an actor
- wants to be in the limelight++

Fastidious++

Case Examples

Attached to his mother++

The first criteria to make friends is their appearance++

"I did not get the partner that I wanted"

- *"I wanted a female with good looks, but my wife is average"*

- *"I got married out of sympathy for her"+++*

Sympathy for the poor+

Was threatened by wife that if he did not get a HIV test done, she would inform his work-place that he has AIDS.

Rubrics in Synthesis Repertory

GENERALS, Food and Drinks, Onions, desire, raw
GENERALS, Food and Drinks, Warm food, desire
GENERALS, Food and Drinks, Fish, aversion
GENERALS, Riding, Car, in a, agg.
HEAD, PAIN, Sun from, exposure
HEAD, PAIN, Sleep, loss of, from late hours
MIND, Delusions, appreciated, he is not
MIND, Homesickness
MIND, Consolation agg.
MIND, Conscientious, trifles about
MIND, Sensitive, opinion of others
MIND, Fear, opinion of others

Prescription : Staphysagaria 1M, II x 2

20/7/98	Erythema >	
	Eruptions dried up	
		CT all
24/7/98	>	
6/10/98	Appetite, thirst- normal	
	Stool, urine- normal	
	No new lesions	
	No oedema of face or legs	CT all
14/11/98	Since 1 month headache twice in a week	
	Pain in eyes, <travelling	
	Nausea, vomiting	
	Grinds teeth at night	SL
22/10/99	Tested HIV+ in June - wife and son also tested +	
	Lost 3kgs in last 3 months	
	Unsatisfactory stools	
	Wife has left him and taken their away son	
	- before marriage he had had sexual affairs with prostitutes	
	Says "I am relieved by my wife leaving me"	
	Speaks of being insulted by friends	

Rubrics

MIND, Delusions, neglected, he is.
MIND, Delusions, insulted, he is
MIND, Longing, good opinion of others
MIND, Consolation agg.
MIND, Fear, insects, of
MIND, Homesickness
GENERALS, Food and Drink, warm food, desires
GENERALS, Food and Drink, fish, aversion

Prescription: Palladium 1M

14/10/99	Vomiting < morning, bilious	
	Vertigo, can't get up from bed	
	< sitting up, > lying	CT all
21/12/99	No complaints	
6/1/00	No complaints	
	Mentally feeling well	
	Appetite normal	
	Sleep normal	
	Stool/ urine normal	CT all
24/1/00	No complaints	CT all
11/2/00	No complaints	S.L.

Case II. 24/11/99

Patient T.A.S.
Female
Married, 3 children
History of Tubercular lymphadenopathy
Family history of TB
    - Tubercular miasm
Possibly infected from blood transfusion 9 years ago

Symptoms

Low grade fever throughout the day
    -during the ninth month of pregnancy
    -with pain in head and shoulders
Child was given up for adoption
Father is HIV -ve
Recurrent apthae in mouth - painless
    - dry feeling in mouth

Weakness in afternoon
Lack of motivation
Vertigo when trying to work, must lie down
Thoughts go through head at night
CD4 290 uL
CD8 1053
Since one week watery coryza
- noseblock
During fever- increased thirst
- desires to lie down
-dullness
- no chill
- no sweat
No appetite
Thirst for 1/2 glass of water at a time
- even though mouth is dry
Perspiration scanty
Tremulous tongue
- yellow posterior coating
Fear of fallin from a height
Cannot tolerate cold weather
Does not admit to problems, says "everything is fine"
Mildness
Does not have good relations with mother-in- law

Rubrics in Synthesis Repertory

GENERALS, Food and Drink, sweets, aversion
MIND, Fear, high places, of
MIND, Quiet, disposition

Case Examples   **199**

    MIND, Asking, nothing for
    MIND, Desires, nothing, desires
    MIND, Hides, true feelings
    MOUTH, Dryness, thirst, with
    EYES, Sunken

Prescription: Arsenicum Album 30c IV x 6

10/1/00   No fever for the last 20 days
        pain in foot
        Bleeding from rectum with stool
            -hard stools
            -anal fissure
        Appetite, thirst normal
        Sleep normal
        Coryza better
        Strength increased- can work again
        Appetite increased   CT all

Case III. 6/1/98

    Patient: Mr. P.A.
    Married with 2 children
    Does not admit or knows how he was infected
    Detected HIV+ 3 years ago
    No presenting complaints
    Family history: Father had diabetes- Tubercular miasm

Symptoms

        Raising phlegm from throat
        < cold water

< cold butter milk
< cold food
Desires sweets+++, Fish++, Chocolate++, Banana+++
Cold foods/ drinks aggravate
Desires cold weather and cold bathing
Fear of water
Nervous when father was sick, felt if he died he would be nowhere
Would like to wear traditional clothing
Responsible
History of alcoholism
Fastidious, things must be in proper place
Sensitive to people's opinion of him
Reserved person
> Consolation
Anxiety over health
Abusive to wife when angry
Suppresses emotions
Avoids talking to strangers
Starting in sleep
Gambles

Rubrics from Synthesis Repertory

GENERALS, Food and Drinks, Cold, drinks, agg.
GENERALS, Food and Drinks, Fish, desires
GENERALS, Food and Drinks, Sweets, desires
MIND, Fastidious

MIND, Reserved
MIND, Company, aversion to, presence of strangers
MIND, Anxiety, family, about his
MIND, Play, gambling, passion for

Prescription: Arsenicum Album 1M, II x 2

4/2/98	No complaints	CT all
5/3/98	No complaints	
	Increased weight	CT all
6/4/98	No complaints	
	Increased weight	CT all
16/4/98	Investigations: CD4 214	
	CD8 2310	
	WBC 5100	
	Hb 15.10	
1/5/98	No complaints	CT all
11/6/98	No complaints	S.L.
29/6/98	Sneezing	S.L.
7/7/98	Sneezing	
	Loss of taste	
	A.A. 10M I x2	
23/7/98	Same	CT all
10/8/98	Investigations: CD4 340	
	CD8 1734	
28/9/98	No complaints	
	Vesicular eruptions on thigh	CT all
17/10/98	Molluscum contagiosum	CT all
7/11/98	No new eruptions	
	No other complaints	CT all
19/11/98	Molluscum on abdomen	CT all
24/12/98	Cold for the last 3 days	
	Watery coryza	CT all
8/1/99	Stool every 2 days	CT all
23/1/99	Investigations: CD4 406	
	CD8 2071	CT all

9/2/99	Coryza- watery	
	-< morning	CT all
25/2/99	Same	CT all
18/5/99	Loose motions 4-5 per day	
	-watery, yellow, with flatulance	CT all
22/6/99	>	
	Hazy vision	
	Left eye pterygium	AA 10M I x2
24/8/99	No complaints	S.L.
23/9/99	CD4 578	
	CD8 2122	
	Evening, eyes feel tired	
	Irritable for the last two months	CT all
25/10/99	No complaints	
28/12/99	No complaints	
28/1/00	No complaints	

■■

Annexure V

HOMOEOPATHY IN INDIA

As early as 1810, missionaries and foreign physicians began distributing homoeopathic medicines in India. However, it was not until 1839 when a Dr. Honigberger from Germany, a student of Hahnemann, was called to Punjab to treat the Maharaja Ranjit Singh, the first official recognition of the healing modality. Several years later, in 1846, Dr. Samuel Brooklyn began the first homoeopathic hospital in India at Tanjore, South India. Until this period, the physicians practicing homoeopathy were predominately from Europe and America, with some teaching going on in private clinics. Some 39 years later, the first homoeopathic college opened its doors in Calcutta, Wes' Bengal, named the Calcutta Homoeopathic Medical College.

Despite the popularity of homoeopathy with the general public due to its cost effectiveness and astounding results, and the enormous amount of qualified homoeopaths practicing throughout India, the government had not yet legislated it until 1937. It was 1937 when a young graduate from the Calcutta Homoeopathic Medical College named Dr. K.G. Saxena approached the Central Legislative Assembly in Delhi with the resolution for homoeopathic recognition. Within a matter of hours, the first major step towards homoeopathic resolution was accomplished. The system could progress as a science and body thus garnering respect and credibility. The resolution was later received by the state governments for consideration allowing the West Bengal government, in 1943, to take the initial steps and constitute the first State Faculty of Homoeopathic Medicine. The All- India Institute of Homoeopathy (in 1980, the name was changed to Indian Institute of Homoeopathic Physicians) was established in 1944 with its head office in Delhi.

In 1962, the Pharmacoepia Committee was formed. This committee prepared the rules and regulations for preparing homoeopathic drugs to be included into the Indian Pharmacoepia. Just one year later the research committee was created. The research committee determined the principles of research in homoeopathy, with an emphasis on the proving of new and old drugs of the materia medica. The committee also decided the subjects of research in various diseases and recommended certain institutions for conducting research. This committee is linked to the present day Central Council for Research in Homoeopathy (CCRH). 1964 saw the creation of the Rural Homoeopathic Medical Aid Committee. This committee considered and recommended how homoeopathy could be implemented towards tackling rural medical problems. As a result of this committee many villages and small town have free government homoeopathic dispensaries.

The aforementioned institute and state faculties allowed the science to thrive and thus create more hospitals and teaching colleges. Due to the explosive growth of teaching facilities, a regulating body was deemed necessary to determine quality of graduates. Thus, in 1974, the then health minister, Dr. Karan Singh, created the Central Council for Homoeopathy in December of the said year. The main functions of the Central Council are: i) to determine minimum standards for granting recognized medical qualifications by medical institutions and universities.

ii) to lay down course and period of study.
iii) to lay down standards for staff, training, equipment, etc.
iv) to frame rules for examinations, examiners, etc.
v) to inspect and regulate colleges.
vi) to maintain a central register of practitioners.
vii) to prescribe standards of professional conduct and code of ethics.
viii) to protect the rights and privileges of practitioners.
viv) to carry out all other matters governing the education and practice of homoeopathy.

Presently, homoeopathic practitioners are required to undertake a degree course of 5 and 1/2 years including internship leading to the degree Bachelor of Homoeopathc Medicine & Surgery. The graduates receive the same level of medical sciences as the equivalent allopathic degree (MBBS). An internship of one year is conducted in a homoeopathic hospital as well as six months internship in an allopathic hospital.

There are presently 125 colleges of homoeopathy in India, 110 of which are attached to state universities. Of which, 6 offer post- graduate M.D. (Hom.) courses of 3 years duration. Each college runs a clinic or a hospital.

Perhaps the best example of a functioning Homoeopathic Hospital would be the Shree Mumbadevi Homoeopathic Hospital and Charitable Trust (See photo 4.3), the teaching hospital of the Smt. Chandaben Mohanbhai Patel (CMP) Homoeopathic Medical College in Mumbai (See photos 4.1 & 4.2). The hospital was established in 1957 by the Homoeopathic Education Society (HES) with the primary objective of promoting and encouraging the science and art of homoeopathy, and to promote the interaction and exchange of ideas between all medical systems.

The medical faculty of the hospital are a combination of homoeopaths and allopaths with a combined effort towards specialties. The hospital runs Out Patient Department (OPD) clinics daily from morning until late afternoon, seeing some 300 patients per day in various departments. The In Patients Department (IPD) and Intensive Cardiac Care Unit (ICCU) has a capacity of 104 beds.

Listing of Various Departments:

Homoeopathy	Gynaecology
Medicine	Research
Paediatrics	Surgery
Rheumatic	ENT
Psychiatric	Orthopaedics
Dental	Ophthalmic
Sonography	Physiotherapy
Plastic Surgery	Radiology
Pathology	Urology
Skin	Cancer

During the years 1998-1999, the various OPDs saw a total of 49'687 patients, whilst 2660 were treated in the IPD and ICCU. The IPD and operating theatres combine homoeopathic with allopathic treatment. The various departments are shared and allopathic and homoeopathic physicians who will assess each case to determine which treatment would be best applied. The operating theatres and ICCU deal primarily in an allopathic surgical setting whilst preoperative and postoperative treatment is done with homoeopathy. ■■

Appendix A

BIBLIOGRAPHY

- Banerjea, S.K. Miasmatic Diagnosis, B. Jain, Delhi, 1992
- Benjamin, E. Immunology: A Short Course, 1991
- Berkow, R. (ed) The Merck Manual, Merck, Rahway, 1992
- Berkow, R. (ed) The Merck Manual, Merck, Rahway, 1999
- CCRH, Rastogi, D.P., et al, Evaluation of homoeopathic therapy in 129 asymptomatic HIV carriers, British Homoeopathic Journal, 1993, 82:4-8
- CCRH, Rastogi, D.P, et al, Homoeopathy in HIV Infection: a trial report of double- blind placebo controlled study, British Homoeopathic Journal, 1999, 88:49-57
- Concorde Coordinating Committee, Concorde MRC/ANRS randomized double-blind controlled trial of immediate vs. Deferred zididuvine in symptom free HIV infection. Lancet. 1994: 343:871-881
- Dahanukar,S. & Thatte, U. Ayurveda Unravelled, National Book Trust, Delhi, 1996
- Dikshit, D. ICR Symposium, Mumbai, Oct. 1999
- Fernandez, I., Migration and HIV/AIDS Vulnerability in South Asia. Presented at the 12th Annual AIDS Conference, Geneva, June- July 1998

- Hahnemann, C.S. The Organon of Medicine, Blaine, Cooper House, 1982
- Kent, J.T. Lectures on Homoeopathic Philosophy, North Atlantic Books, Berkeley, 1995
- Koehler, G., Ler rbuch der homoopatie, Hippokratis Verlag GmbH, Stuttgart, 1983
- Koehler, G. The Handbook of Homoeopathy: Its principle and practice, Healing Arts Press, Rochester, 1989
- Master, F. Bedside Organon of Medicine, B. Jain, Delhi, 1994
- Master, F. Homoeopathic Dictionary of Dreams, B. Jain, Delhi, 1999
- Master, F. Perceiving Rubrics of the Mind, B. Jain, Delhi, 1992
- Master, F. Sycotic Shame, B. Jain, Delhi, 1994
- Master, F. Tubercular Miasm Tuberculins, B. Jain, Delhi, 1997
- Roberts, H. The Principles and Art of Cure by Homooopathy, B. Jain, Delhi, 1995
- Scholtan, J. Homoeopathy and the Elements, Hompath Software, Mumbai, 1999
- Shah, C. P. Public Health and Preventive Medicine in Canada, UofT, Toronto, 1999, 4th ed.
- Sterlick, J. AIDS: The Homoeopathic Challenge, Dove, London, 1996
- Strange, M., Communication, February 1999, London
- Strange, M. AIDS- Some early clinical experiences, British Homoeopathic Journal, 1988, 77:224-227
- Vithoulkas, G. Materia Medica Viva, Health and Habitat, Mill Valley, 1992

Bibliography

- Volberding, P.A., et al, A comparison of immediate with deferred Zididuvine therapy for asymptomatic HIV infected adults with CD4 cell counts of 500 or more per cubic mm. New England Journal of Medicine, 1995, 333: 408- 413
- Werner, D., & Bower.B. Helping Health Workers Learn, Hesperian, Berkeley, 1999
- Werner, D. Where there is no doctor: a village health care handbook, Hesperian, Berkeley, 1999

Appendix B

ENDNOTES

[i] Shah, C. **Public Health and Preventive Medicine in Canada,** UofT Press, Toronto, 1998, 4th edt.

[ii] Singh,D. **Understanding AIDS**, Delhi, 1996, National Book Trust

[iii] Pawar, S. Personal Interview, October 4,1999, Mumbai

[iv] Shah, C. **Public Health and Preventive Medicine in Canada**, UofT Press, Toronto, 1998, 4th edt.

[v] AIDS and HIV in Canada HIV / AIDS Epidemic Update, Bureau of HIV/AIDS, STD and TB Update Series, Laboratory Centre for Disease Control, May 1999 ,

www.hc-sc.gc.ca/hpb/lcdc/bah/epi/ahcan-_e.html

[vi] McMurray, A. **Community Health and Wellness: a Socioecological Approach**, page 31, Mosby, Artarmon, 1999,

[vii] Shah, C., page 208, **Public Health and Preventive Medicine in Canada**, UofT Press, Toronto, 1998, 4th edt.

[viii] Ransen K. Personal Interview, Oct. 2, 99, Anand, Gujarat

[ix] Christian, S. Personal Interview, September 18,1999, Anand, Gujarat

[x] Shah, C., page 208, **Public Health and Preventive Medicine in Canada**, UofT Press, Toronto, 1998, 4th edt.

[xi] Park, **Textbook of Preventive and Social Medicine**, 17th edt., Delhi, 1998

[xii] Ibid

[xiii] Berkow, R.(ed) **Merck Manual**, Rahway, 1992, Merck

[xiv] Park, **Textbook of Preventive and Social Medicine**, 17th edt., Delhi, 1998

[xv] International Journal of Health Education, June 1993, Vol. XII/2,P.S.

[xvi] UNAIDS/WHO, Website, www.unaids.org/hivaidsinfo/statistics/

[xvii] Horowitz, L. Total Health Seminar, June 1999, Toronto

[xviii] Singh, D., page28, **Understanding AIDS**, Delhi, 1996, National Book Trust

[xix] Ibid

[xx] Ibid

[xxi] Korber, B. Los Almos National Laboratory, website, www.timesofindia.com/050200/05hlth13/htm

[xxii] British Medical Journal, 1992, 304:809-813

[xxiii] Park, **Textbook of Preventive and Social Medicine**, 17th edt., Delhi, 1998

[xxiv] Ibid, page 240

[xxv] Ibid

[xxvi] UNAIDS/WHO, Website, www.unaids.org/hivaidsinfo/statistics/june98/fact_sheets/pdfs/india.pdf

[xxvii] Shah, C., **Public Health and Preventive Medicine in Canada**, UofT Press, Toronto, 1998, 4th edt.

[xxviii] UNAIDS/WHO, Website, www.unaids.org/hivaidsinfo/statistics/june98/fact_sheets/pdfs/india.pdf

[xxix] Gilada, I.S. **AIDS ASIA** (Journal, IHO) Mumbai, issue 3, May, 1999

[xxx] Christian, S., Personal Interview, September 18,1999, Anand, Gujarat

[xxxi] Berkow, R. (ed) , **Merck Manual**, Rahway, 1992, Merck

[xxxii] Park, **Textbook of Preventive and Social Medicine**, 17th edt., Delhi, 1998

[xxxiii] Ibid

[xxxiv] Ibid

[xxxv] Singh, V. CCRH, Personal Conversation, August 9, 1999, Mumbai

[xxxvi] Berkow, R.(ed), **Merck Manual**, Rahway, 1992, Merck

[xxxvii] Shah, C., page 211, **Public Health and Preventive Medicine in Canada**, UofT Press, Toronto, 1998, 4th edt.

[xxxviii] Christian, S., Personal Interview, September 18,1999, Anand, Gujarat

[xxxix] Regunathan, S. Health India: HIV/AIDS Fear Feeds on Myths. Website www.oneworld.org/ips2/june98/13_12_043.html

[xl] Ibid

[xli] Epstein, D. , WHO Report, World Health Assembly, 1999, Geneva

[xlii] Park, **Textbook of Preventive and Social Medicine**, 17th edt., Delhi, 1998

[xliii] Berkow, R. (ed), page 78, **Merck Manual**, Rahway, 1992, Merck

[xliv] Gilada, I.S. **AIDS ASIA** Journal, IHO, Mumbai, Issue 3, May 1999

[xlv] Christian, S., Personal Interview, September 18,1999, Anand, Gujarat

[xlvi] Park, , **Textbook of Preventive and Social Medicine**, 17th edt., Delhi, 1998

[xlvii] Ibid

[xlviii] Christian, S., Personal Interview, September 18,1999, Anand, Gujarat

[xlix] Rao, M.R. **AIDS ACTION**, " Tracking the Trucks", Asia Pacific edt., Issue 40, July- Sept., 1998, Quezon City

[l] Tan, M. **AIDS ACTION**, Asia- Pacific edt. Issue 40, July- Sept. 1998, Quezon City

[li] Fernandez, I. **Migration and HIV/AIDS Vulnerability in South East Asia**, presented at the 12th annual AIDS Conference in Geneva, June- July, 1998

[lii] Rao, M.R., **AIDS ACTION**, " Tracking the Trucks", Asia Pacific edt., Issue 40, July- Sept., 1998, Quezon City

[liii] Pawar, S., HIV Unit Coordinator, Mumbai, Personal Interview, Oct 26, 1999

[liv] Park, **Textbook of Preventive and Social Medicine**, 17th edt., Delhi, 1998

[lv] Christian, S., Personal Interview, September 18,1999, Anand, Gujarat

[lvi] Ibid

[lvii] Ibid

[lviii] Christopher, S., Emery Hospital Administrator, Personal Interview, Oct.4, 1999

[lix] Ibid

[lx] Davidson, N. **AIDS ACTION**, "A Better Life and Death" Asia- Pacific edt., Issue 41, Oct- Dec., 1998, Quezon City

Endnotes 215

[lxi] Shah, J., Paediatric Surgeon, Personal Interview, Oct. 21, 1999, Vadodara, Gujarat, India

[lxii] Dave, P.C., Homoeopath, Personal Interview, Oct. 21, 1999, Vadodara, Gujarat, India

[lxiii] Public Health Billboard, Anand, Gujarat

[lxiv] Christian, S., Emery Hospital Administrator, Personal Interview, Oct.4, 1999

[lxv] Berkow, R. (ed), **Merck Manual**, Rahway, 1992, Merck

[lxvi] Ruparil, P. Pharmacist, Personal Conversation, Sept. 29, 1999, Porbandar, Gujarat

[lxvii] Dave, P.C., Homoeopath, Personal Interview, Oct. 21, 1999, Vadodara, Gujarat, India

[lxviii] Hospet Express, December 3, 1999

[lxix] Hospet Express, Ibid

[lxx] Tan, M. **AIDS Action** *"Migration and Risk"*, Asia Pacific etd., Issue 40, July- Sept., 1998, Quezon City

[lxxi] Southeast Asian J Trop Med Public Health. 1998 Jun;29(2):373-6. Unique Identifier : AIDSLINE MED/99101222

Misra SN; Sengupta D; Satpathy SK; National AIDS Control Organization, New Delhi, India.

[lxxii] Gilada, I.S., **AIDS ASIA** Journal, IHO, Mumbai, Issue 3, May 1999

[lxxiii] Herdt, G. **Sexual Cultures and Population Movement: Implications for AIDS/STD's**, Oxford, Oxford University Press, 1997

[lxxiv] Gilada, I.S., **AIDS ASIA** Journal, IHO, Mumbai, Issue 3, May 1999

[lxxv] Jain, K., Homoeopath, Personal Interview, Oct. 20, 1999, Vadodara, Gujarat

[lxxvi] National AIDS Control Oganization (NACO), www.naco.nic.in/vsnaco/indiascene/indscen.htm

[lxxvii] Panicker, L.Times of India, **A Positive Strategy: Gender Discrimination in HIV/AIDS Epidemic**, Oct, 26, 1999

[lxxviii] Singh, D. Ibid

[lxxix] National AIDS Control Oganization (NACO), www.naco.nic.in/vsnaco/indiascene/indscen.htm

[lxxx] Times of India, **AIDS Day**, December 1, 1999

[lxxxi] Baker, A., Fox, K., de Groot,C., Honan,N. Homoeopathic Links, volume 8, 1995, 2/95, Asian edt.

[lxxxii] Solomon, G.F., "Psychoneuroimmunology and Human Immunodeficiency virus Infection" Psych. Med. Vol. 2

[lxxxiii] 'Raju', Personal Interview, Oct. 29, 1999, Mumbai

[lxxxiv] Salvation Army, Mumbai HIV/AIDS Community Development **Home Care** Booklet, 1999

[lxxxv] Physicians Desk Reference, Medical Economics Corporation, 1997

[lxxxvi] Ibid

[lxxxvii] Concorde Coordinating Committee. Concorde MRC/ANRS randomized double-blind controlled trial of immediate vs. deferred zididuvine in symptom free HIV infection. Lancet. 1994:343:871-881

[lxxxviii] British Medical Research Council and the French National AIDS Research Agency (Concorde Group), **The Concorde Study**, aegis.com/pubs/gmhc/1993/GM070401.htm

[lxxxix] Volberding PA, Lagakos SW, Grimes JM, et al. The duration of zidovudine benefit in persons with asymptomatic HIV infection: prolonged evaluation of protocol 019 of the AIDS Clinical Trials Group. JAMA 1994;272:437–42.

[xc] Hahnemann, C.S., **Organon of Medicine**, Blaine, 1982, Cooper Publishing

[xci] Rastogi, D.P., Singh, V.P., Singh, V. Dey, K.**The British Homoeopathic Journal, Evaluation of homoeopathc therapy in 129 asymptomatic HIV carriers** CCRH, January, 1993, Vol. 82, pp. 4-8

[xcii] Rastogi, D.P. et al **Homeopathy in HIV infection: a trial report of double-blind placebo controlled study**, British Homoeopathic Journal (1999)88, 49-57, Stockton Press

[xciii] Ibid

[xciv] Robert W. Doms, Aimee L. Edinger, and John P. Moore, Coreceptor Use by Primate Lentiviruses, http//hiv-web.lanl.gov/HTML/reviews/Doms98.html

[xcv] Marcos E. Garcia-Ojeda, ACT UP, T-Cell receptors CCR5 and CXCR4,www.actupgg.org/BAR/art062696.html

[xcvi] Moore, JP. Coreceptors: Implications for HIV Pathogenesis and Therapy. Science. 1997:272:51-52

[xcvii] Little, D., The Origin of Homeo-prophylaxis, www.similimum.com/Thelittlelibrairy/Homeopathicphilosophy/prohylaxis.html

[xcviii] "Tony", Personal Interview, Oct. 29, 1999, Mumbai

[xcix] Hahnemann, C.S. **Organon of Medicine**, Blaine, 1982, Cooper Pub. Aphorism 78

[c] Shah, J. **Hompath Classic**, user guide, Hompath, 1999, Mumbai

[ci] Banerjea, S.K. **Miasmatic Diagnosis**, Delhi, 1992, B.Jain

[cii] Ibid

[ciii] ilbid

[civ] Ibid